LANCE ARMSTRONG

LANCE ARMSTRONG

A Biography

Paula Johanson

GREENWOOD BIOGRAPHIES

GREENWOOD

AN IMPRINT OF ABC-CLIO, LLC
Santa Barbara, California • Denver, Colorado • Oxford, England

Library of Congress Cataloging-in-Publication Data

Johanson, Paula.
  Lance Armstrong : a biography / Paula Johanson.
    p. cm. — (Greenwood biographies)
  Includes bibliographical references and index.
    ISBN 978-0-313-38690-9 (hardback) — ISBN 978-0-313-38691-6
(ebook)   1. Armstrong, Lance.   2. Cyclists—United States—
Biography.   3. Cancer—Patients—United States—Biography.
4. Tour de France (Bicycle race)—History.   I. Title.
  GV1051.A76J65 2011
  796.6'2092—dc22
  [B]   2010051150

ISBN: 978-0-313-38690-9
EISBN: 978-0-313-38691-6

15 14 13 12 11   1 2 3 4 5

This book is also available on the World Wide Web as an eBook.
Visit www.abc-clio.com for details.

Greenwood
An Imprint of ABC-CLIO, LLC

ABC-CLIO, LLC
130 Cremona Drive, P.O. Box 1911
Santa Barbara, California 93116-1911

This book is printed on acid-free paper ∞

Manufactured in the United States of America

For my friends John and Louise, who go biking and kayaking with me and keep me writing books.

CONTENTS

SERIES FOREWORD

In response to high school and public library needs, Greenwood developed this distinguished series of full-length biographies specifically for student use. Prepared by field experts and professionals, these engaging biographies are tailored for high school students who need challenging yet accessible biographies. Ideal for secondary school assignments, the length, format and subject areas are designed to meet educators' requirements and students' interests.

Greenwood offers an extensive selection of biographies spanning all curriculum-related subject areas including social studies, the sciences, literature and the arts, history and politics, as well as popular culture, covering public figures and famous personalities from all time periods and backgrounds, both historic and contemporary, who have made an impact on American and/or world culture. Greenwood biographies were chosen based on comprehensive feedback from librarians and educators. Consideration was given to both curriculum relevance and inherent interest. The result is an intriguing mix of the well known and the unexpected, the saints and sinners from long-ago history and contemporary pop culture. Readers will find a wide array of subject choices from fascinating crime figures like Al Capone to inspiring pioneers like Margaret Mead, from the greatest minds of our time like Stephen Hawking to the most amazing success stories of our day like J. K. Rowling.

While the emphasis is on fact, not glorification, the books are meant to be fun to read. Each volume provides in-depth information about the subject's life from birth through childhood, the teen years, and adulthood. A thorough account relates family background and education, traces personal and professional influences, and explores struggles, accomplishments, and contributions. A timeline highlights the most significant life events against a historical perspective. Bibliographies supplement the reference value of each volume.

INTRODUCTION

The hum of a bicycle's wheels on pavement is a subtle, attractive sound. It's a siren call that Lance Armstrong has heard since he was a small child growing up in Dallas, Texas. When a dozen or more riders race their bikes together, that siren call grows even more powerful. The hum of bicycle wheels has dominated Lance Armstrong's life as he has become one of the world's top-ranked professional cyclists. When he was ill with testicular cancer, as long as he was riding a bicycle he could tell himself he was still alive. While still recovering from cancer treatment, Armstrong rode in a charity bike event, a fund-raiser to launch the Lance Armstrong Foundation. After his illness he made an amazing comeback to professional racing, taking a bronze medal at the Sydney Olympics. Armstrong won the most challenging race in the world, the Tour de France, seven times in a row before retiring. At age 37, he made a second comeback. His goal was to use his professional cycling to promote cancer awareness worldwide through the Lance Armstrong Foundation.

Lance Edward Armstrong was born Lance Edward Gunderson on September 1, 1971, in Dallas, Texas. His parents, Linda Mooneyham and Eddie Gunderson, divorced while he was still a baby. His mother's second husband, Terry Armstrong, adopted young Lance and gave him his name. Lance kept that name—Armstrong—after his mother's second divorce and made it his own. As hard work brought them improved living conditions, their little family moved from housing projects in Oak Cliff, a run-down suburb of Dallas, to a nice apartment in Richardson and a house in Plano. The energetic boy was riding a toddler's toy tricycle on his second birthday and a tuned-up secondhand bike for play before he was six. Lance rode the school bus to public elementary, middle, and high school. At least, he rode the bus until scuffling fights with classmates got him booted off, and after that he bicycled to school. His mother gave him good bikes when he showed an interest in BMX racing and triathlons. The investment paid off. Before graduating from high school, her son had sponsors and his own car bought with prize money. He didn't go on to college as many of his school friends did. His career as a world-class cyclist was launched.

By his 25th birthday, Armstrong was confident in his place in the world. He had new corporate sponsors and had just signed a two-year contract with a new team, Cofidis. His girlfriend was beautiful and smart. The new house he'd just built in Austin, Texas, had a Porsche in the driveway and fine art on the walls. All of that was shaken to the core by unexpected news: he had testicular cancer. It was not just a single tumor that might take years to affect his health. The very day that his cancer was diagnosed, he was too sore to ride a bike. Tumors had already spread to his abdomen and lungs. A few days later, a skilled surgeon lifted off the top of his skull like the lid of a Halloween pumpkin so that two more tumors could be removed.

As Armstrong finished treatment for cancer, he resolved to start a charitable foundation. The Lance Armstrong Foundation started out small but with a lot of hope and ambition. There were many volunteers before any employee was hired. Funds were donated by both large corporations and smaller business sponsors. Since 1997, the Lance Armstrong Foundation has raised over $260 million in charitable donations. The funds are used to sponsor cancer research and to support people with cancer.

Much of Armstrong's life is reported by journalists in print, on television, and on Internet Web sites. Armstrong has tried not to let his life revolve around publicity. Press releases and Web sites for the Lance

Armstrong Foundation promote many other riders and cancer survivors, not him alone. His home life has become very precious to him after a divorce, a broken engagement, and a series of shorter relationships. He is the proud father of five children. Concern for the needs of his children is his first priority as he looks to the future.

His three older children were born during his first comeback to professional racing. After recovering from cancer, he was not only a strong rider but an effective member of a racing team. Armstrong doesn't believe he would ever have won the Tour de France without the support of his teammates. He retired in part because his children wanted him to travel less and be at home more. His younger children were born during his second comeback. This time around, as he travels for cycling and for the Lance Armstrong Foundation, he is taking care to keep the family bonds strong.

Surviving cancer may have been the hardest challenge Armstrong has had to face. Another challenge that he's faced for years is being accused of using banned performance-enhancing drugs. Since he was a teenager winning triathlons competing against trained adults, he has been accused of using drugs. As he returned to cycling after his cancer treatment, the accusations started again. Test after test has shown no signs that Armstrong has ever used methods or drugs banned by the International Cycling Union (Union Cycliste Internationale, or UCI). He is one of the most tested athletes in the world.

September is the start of the new year for most people in school, and September 2008 was the start of a new time in Armstrong's life. At age 37, he announced that he would return to professional cycling for a second comeback. His purpose was to raise global awareness about cancer. There would be increased publicity about his athletic competition, now that he was no longer a young hotshot. This increased attention would bring more international awareness to the Lance Armstrong Foundation and its many programs supporting people living with cancer. However, many commentators believe that he had another intent as well: to dispel once and for all the claims about his using performance-enhancing drugs.

There were certainly many chances to prove or dispel these claims. From 2008 to 2010, many dozens of drug tests were performed on Armstrong's urine and blood. He passed every test. Armstrong also had many chances to promote awareness of how cancer affects the lives of over 28 million people around the world. The Lance Armstrong Foundation has many programs to support individuals and sponsor cancer research. Armstrong met with elected officials and spoke at charity events in many countries.

At this point in his life, Armstrong may be at the end of his career as a professional cyclist. He is already older than most of his fellow riders. Some of his rivals in 2010 were the sons of men Armstrong had raced against in his own youth. He is hardly at the end of his life, though. It is possible that he can look forward to not just many years of supporting his foundation and his community, but decades. As a businessman and an investor, Armstrong is taking an interest in city planning. He hasn't ruled out a possible political career in the future. And it is certain that he is hoping to be the good father his growing children need him to be.

TIMELINE: EVENTS IN THE LIFE OF LANCE ARMSTRONG

1971 Born September 18, 1971, named Lance Edward Gunderson

1974 Legally adopted by Terry Armstrong

1989 Competes in the World Junior Cycling Championships in Moscow
Graduates high school
Joins the U.S. national cycling team

1992 Olympics in Barcelona; places 14th in the road race
Joins the Motorola cycling team as a professional
Finishes last in first professional race, Clásica de San Sebastián, Spain

1993 Wins the World Road Race championship in Oslo, Norway

1996 Considered the seventh-ranked cyclist in the world
Wins the Tour DuPont in North Carolina
Competes in Olympics in Atlanta, Georgia, placing 6th in the time trial and 12th in the road race
October 2: Cancer diagnosis

October through December: chemotherapy, surgeries, and more chemotherapy

1997 February: Cancer-free
Launches the Lance Armstrong Foundation
Gets engaged to Kristin Richard

1998 Returns to competitive cycling
Marries Kristin Richard

1999 Wins the Tour de France
First child, Luke Armstrong, born

2000 Wins the Tour de France

2001 Wins the Tour de France
Twin daughters, Grace and Isabella Armstrong, born

2002 Wins the Tour de France

2003 Wins the Tour de France
Divorces Kristin Richard

2004 Wins the Tour de France

2005 Wins the Tour de France
Gets engaged to Sheryl Crow

2006 Breaks engagement to Sheryl Crow
Pace car driver for the Indianapolis 500

2007 Founds charity foundation, Athletes for Hope

2008 Meets girlfriend Anna Hansen
September: Announces return to professional cycling at age 37

2009 Fourth child, Max Armstrong, born to Anna Hansen
Places third in the Tour de France

2010 Finishes Tour de France
Fifth child, Olivia Armstrong, born to Anna Hansen

Chapter 1

A UNIQUE CYCLIST

Lance Armstrong believes that each of us makes choices every day. "The way you live your life, the perspective you select, is a choice you make every single day when you wake up," he said in his 2003 memoir, *Every Second Counts*. "It's yours to decide."[1] The choices he has made have led him around the world. He has ridden his bike in professional races and also for relaxation. His bike has kept moving on a variety of road surfaces and in all kinds of weather. He's been celebrated in front of crowds, and he's been scolded by cycling mentors that he trusts.

In high school, Armstrong had friends from different social circles. Some were into sports, though few had the focused attitude that he had. Others had plans to go on to college, where they would study or party. One of his friends, Lee Walker, liked to quote the poet Mary Oliver: "Tell me, what is it you plan to do with your one wild and precious life?"[2] Even then, Armstrong knew he was born to ride hard.

AGGRESSIVE RIDER

As a cyclist, Armstrong has not been shy in showing his emotions. The aggressive style of his riding has been consistent since he was an amateur. It took a lot of insistent coaching from Chris Carmichael to convince him that charging to the front of the pack for the entire race was not the best way to ride. Even after he learned to ride tactically, Armstrong would cross the finish line with a great show of emotion. Dozens of photographs show Armstrong winning races and raising his fists to the sky, shouting or even screaming in triumph.

As he became the first winner in 1993 of the Thrift Drug Classic, the Triple Crown of American cycling, he did a little grandstanding. When finishing the third race, the U.S. professional cycling national championship, he had a big enough lead to blow his mother a kiss. He sat up on his bike during the final lap, took out a comb, and ran it through his hair. He smiled for the cameras and the Philadelphia crowds. He was 21 years old, and he had just won a million-dollar prize. The moment was worth a little showing off. He finished with the biggest margin of victory that had ever been recorded for that race. And he was the first rider ever to win that prize.

Winning that Triple Crown meant winning a one-day race in Pittsburgh and a six-day stage race in West Virginia before competing in a 156-mile race through Philadelphia at the U.S. pro championship. Armstrong had to show talents usually developed in riders who are sprinters, or climbers who can ride up hills, or stage racers who can make a supreme effort day after day in changing terrain. He had to learn to be consistent instead of just charging ahead from the start.

DANGEROUS LIFESTYLE

Growing up energetic and reckless, Armstrong was a no-holds-barred competitor as an amateur. With careful coaching from Chris Carmichael, he emerged in his early twenties as a powerful professional ranked among the world's best cyclists. He has raced on cobblestone roads in the rain, among two dozen or more other riders, with motorcycles right behind them and crowds an arm's length away. He has trained on the mountain roads of France, Spain, and Italy in all kinds of weather, from baking heat to sleet and snow, weeks before races would take place. He has survived collisions and injuries that could have ended any rider's life, let alone his career. One horrifying crash on a lonely mountain road broke his neck. But that incident didn't convince him to slow down, in or out of competition.

"The craziest and most dangerous thing I do these days is argue with truckers," Armstrong wrote in *Every Second Counts*. "Over the years, I've been run off the road by too many pickups and rock trucks to count. Texas truck drivers hate cyclists; we have an ongoing war with them on the state byways. I've been blown into ditches, hit by stones, and threatened with tire irons."[3]

MELLOW JOHNNY'S BIKE STORE

One of the things that has brought Armstrong great satisfaction is opening his own bicycle store. He believes that everyone can and should ride a bike. Based in Austin, it's a bike store for local riders, not just for elite international competitors. One sign of that inclusiveness is the name of the store: Mellow Johnny's Bike Shop. For customers looking for a fine big store where they can see a good range of bikes, that just sounds like a name with a good attitude. But for customers who know that owner Lance Armstrong has won the Tour de France many times, it's an inside joke.

The leader of each day's stage in the Tour de France wears a yellow jersey during the next day's stage. The yellow shirt is also worn by the overall winner. Armstrong has worn the yellow jersey so many times that many people think of him in yellow shirts. After all, that's how he's shown in sports magazines and news photographs and videos, winning races. The French words for "yellow jersey" are *maillot jaune*. Try to say that in English! It sounds a little like "mah yoh zhone." "Mellow Johnny" is about as close as an English speaker can get. That's what the British riders call the man wearing the yellow jersey.

When an American rider started making such a good name for himself at the 1999 Tour de France, American journalists started paying more attention to this race. They tried to learn the lingo and make good news reports about this sport. "Mellow Johnny" is one of the terms they picked up and made popular. It makes a good name for a bike store, and it really does show a good attitude. This isn't a store named for a famous athlete. This store is named for the shirt that many winners have worn. And it's named for a nickname, not a fussy, precise word in another language. Often in 2009 and 2010, when booking into a hotel while on a riding tour, Armstrong registered using the name "Johnny Mellow." He also rode on the Tour of the Gila with his friends Levi Leipheimer and Chris Horner as a team called "The Mellow Johnnys."

Armstrong, his employees, and his friends all try to make this bike shop a center for the cycling community in Austin. "To serve the bike community is our job," says the Mellow Johnny's Bike Store Web site, "but to convert people to a bike life is our mission."[4] As well as bikes and equipment for sale, the store has a service department and repair shop.

Something special here that most bike stores don't have is a section with showers, lockers, and bike storage that people can rent for a dollar a day. The owner of this shop wants people commuting to work to know about this place and use it and to participate in the fitness and social activities that happen here. A place to clean up after a ride is important, especially for commuters going to work. Lockers for riding clothes and safe bike storage simply aren't available at most people's workplaces. This element of the store shows Armstrong's background. He was never only a competitor in races and nothing else. Through his teen years and as an adult, he rode his bike every day. He rode to school, to friends' homes, and to sports practices. That's how he got around. Arriving somewhere covered in sweat is something he knows all about. He also knows what it feels like to have a bike stolen.

Armstrong goes for long rides even when he's not training, day after day. He gets bored riding the same route over and over. Changing his routes helps, and sometimes, so does having friends along for the ride. The store hosts rides at a variety of experience levels, along routes that change all the time. The summer activity schedule for the store shows events five days a week. The employees also teach people how to maintain their bikes, changing flat tires and so on. There are even yoga classes to help cyclists wind down after a long ride. The result is a store that is trying to bring to many people in Austin the good feeling of having bikes in their lives. Having bikes has made Armstrong and his friends well and healthy, and they want to share that feeling.

FATHERHOOD

Becoming a father was an achievement that changed Armstrong's life completely. His attitudes about winning and competing, his fears of losing or being unable to compete—these all took second place to being a father.

His three older children, Luke, Isabella, and Grace, love receiving mail from abroad. When he's traveling in other countries, Armstrong takes the time to write to them. Postcards take only a few minutes and give a real sense of connection. When he is traveling, the family also uses computers and webcams for internet chats, something that pleases all of them.

Though they are now divorced, Armstrong and his ex-wife, Kristin Richards Armstrong, are working hard to maintain a strong sense of family for their children. Their homes in Austin are only a few minutes apart. When Armstrong is at home in Austin, he lives with his girl-friend, Anna Hansen, and their two young children, Max and Olivia. He's usually the parent who drives Luke, Isabella, and Grace to school. After dropping them off, he goes for a long training ride, and then he picks up the kids after school is over.

For Armstrong's eldest child, Luke, one of the most important races of the year is not a bike race, it's the Pinewood Derby. The competitors are youngsters who build model cars out of a block of pine, then race them. It's a father-and-son project for young Luke and his dad. Over a couple of months, they consult with experts for design ideas. Luke ends up doing most of the designing himself, as well as sanding the model and attaching the wheels. There are strict rules about the model cars, including the required weight of exactly five ounces (142 grams). Armstrong takes real pride in his son's third-place finish in the 2009 derby.

There are young cousins in Armstrong's family, the children of his mother's brother and sisters. He's glad to keep up a connection with them at various weddings and other family gatherings. His mother is a doting grandparent. There is no ongoing contact between Armstrong and the families of either his birth father or his adoptive father.

What he needs from a father, Armstrong has been lucky enough to be given by sports mentors such as J. T. Hoyt, Jim Ochowicz, and Eddy Merckx. "Always nice to have a visit from the greatest cyclist of all time," Armstrong says of Merckx. "I'm so grateful for the way he's taken me under his wing."[5]

Armstrong has no nieces or nephews of his own, but there are some young people he has been close to for all their young lives. One of these is Marco Casartelli, son of Fabio Casartelli. In 1995, Armstrong and Fabio Casartelli were teammates on the U.S. Postal Services cycling team. During the Tour de France, Casartelli was in a horrible crash and died from his injuries. Just a month earlier, Fabio and Annalisa Casartelli had celebrated the birth of their son, Marco. Armstrong has kept in touch with Annalisa and Marco ever since. A couple of times, Marco has interviewed him for school projects.

EATING LIKE A KID

While many children like to eat sweet things, it's common for adults to lose that sweet tooth as they mature. Not Armstrong! For breakfast he often eats a lot of carbohydrates for quick energy. For the last dozen years or more, that's usually a bowl of muesli and some fruit. He burns off more calories during five hours of riding his bike than most people need to eat in an entire day. On his bread every morning, instead of peanut butter he takes Nutella, a sweet spread made from hazelnuts, milk, and cocoa powder that's very popular among European cyclists.

During cold and wet days of racing and training, he reaches for a candy bar. The sugars in it are quickly digested, giving his blood sugar a boost and increasing available energy. "On an otherwise miserable day, nothing lifts my spirits like a Snickers bar,"[6] he admitted in his third memoir, *Comeback 2.0*. A candy bar may not be the lunch of champions, but it does the trick of getting him through a cold day. At dinner, he is careful to eat a healthy meal. During the 2009 Tour of California, there were many cold and rainy days. He enjoyed eating pizza in his hotel room after those hard days on the bike. Sometimes pizza or candy bars are comfort food. Tex-Mex food, such as burritos, is a treat for him.

Aside from sweet things eaten as fuel, the majority of what Armstrong eats can be called health food. Since he was a boy, he always ate a reasonably balanced diet of home-cooked food. As a young man, he began a lifelong enjoyment of Shriner Bock beer and Tex-Mex food. When he was diagnosed with cancer, a nutritionist recommended that he eat organically raised chicken and fresh fruits and vegetables and avoid junk food. For the most part, more than 12 years later he still keeps to a healthy diet of mostly natural foods. Straying from this diet can be cause for regret. During the 2010 cycling season, he had to drop out of three races because of gastroenteritis, which may have been due to what he ate.

TOURING CALIFORNIA

In February 2009, huge crowds turned out to cheer on the riders in the Tour of California. Armstrong rode on the Mellow Johnny's team. This is a race over many days, done in multiple stages like the Tour de France. Some stages take cyclists through hills and valleys, and there are time trials. The fifth stage takes the riders through the Central Valley and its groves of flowering almond trees. Every January and February, hives of bees are brought to this valley from all over the United States to pollinate the flowering trees. In 2009 the hives were suffering catastrophic losses of bees, for reasons not fully understood. The health and vigor of Armstrong and the other riders passing through this valley was a good omen for the people of this region, who depend on the vigor of their visitors, whether bees or athletes.

For the crowds, there were many heroes competing, not only Armstrong. Some of these men have become Armstrong's friends as well as his colleagues and competitors. The winner in 2009 was Armstrong's friend and training partner, Levi Leipheimer. It was Leipheimer's third consecutive win of the Tour of California.

This state is not all beaches and farmland valleys. One of the longest, toughest climbs of the Tour of California takes the riders up Palomar Mountain. At the top of this mountain, 1,700 meters (about 5,600 feet) high, is Mount Palomar Observatory. Here astronomers study the solar system as well as near and distant stars. One research program keeps track of asteroids whose paths come close to Earth. For years, scientists at the observatory have made historically important discoveries.

Armstrong has personal history on Mount Palomar, too, dating back to 1986. As a young man he lived with friends in San Diego for a summer, training as a triathlete. Most of the training rides he took at that time brought him up that mountain. It takes two hours to drive from downtown San Diego up to the observatory, which makes it a decent ride for Armstrong. It had been 20 years since he'd last been there. Going back to Mount Palomar in 2009 was a landmark on his second comeback, a clear sign that he was not only in good form but in touch with his past as well.

IN TOUCH WITH FANS

It's important for celebrities to allow some information about themselves to be available to fans. Whether he likes it or not, Armstrong is as notable a celebrity as he is a competitive cyclist. And he does seem to like some of the attention he gets from fans and journalists. There has been a Web site maintained for him for years. The content of the Web site is as much about the Lance Armstrong Foundation as it is about Armstrong's own activities. As social media such as Facebook and Twitter became popular, Armstrong began making posts to a circle of fans.

The Twitter fans were useful in 2009 when Armstrong's cycling team had some bikes go missing. "A few of our bikes were stolen from the back of the team truck while we were in Sacramento, including the bike I use for time trials," Armstrong wrote in *Comeback 2.0*. The police were notified. Officers came to interview the mechanics and team directors, and to take fingerprints from the truck. Armstrong had 100,000 Twitter followers at that time. "I put up what amounted to an APB for the stolen goods. In the end, we got the bikes back and the suspects were apprehended—through the efforts of the Sacramento Police Department."[7] Armstrong's bike was missing for only four days before someone brought it anonymously to a police station.

These thousands of Twitter followers were not only helpful in the case of the stolen bikes. They also had an opportunity to show their sensible natures. At one point, Armstrong wrote a phone message containing his personal phone number and accidentally sent it out on Twitter to all of his followers. Surprisingly few people took advantage of knowing his phone number. He did end up changing the phone number to regain some control over his privacy.

MET IN PASSING

What's it like for a bicyclist who looks over at the rider coming up from behind to pass, and realizes that it's Lance Armstrong? Many amateur riders have met Armstrong for a few seconds, or a minute, or a few miles on a training ride. By all reports, for them the meeting is a bright moment in what is often a lonely and tiring sport.

One of these brief meetings was caught on film in January 2009 on the big island of Hawaii. "Every day in Hawaii I saw this cyclist in the pink top," Armstrong said in *Comeback 2.0*. "I'd give her a little wave; she'd wave back."[8]

Armstrong wasn't just girl-watching as he passed some hot young babe. This cyclist was not a slim, hard-bodied athlete; a photo taken by his friend Elizabeth Kreutz shows the cyclist as a woman in her middle years. Instead of gear resembling Armstrong's technical sport shirt and bike shorts, she is wearing a black beach-wrap skirt tied over a pink bikini. Her flip-flop sandals seem to grip her bike's pedals adequately without need for the clip-on shoes that professional bikers wear.

There's a strong visual contrast in Kreutz's photo. One rider is a lean man tipped forward on a racing bike with his corded muscles bulging. The other rider is a relaxed woman sitting upright on a cruiser with her rounded limbs in motion. Both riders look so mobile, so active. It's obvious that both are enjoying their ride along the same stretch of road surrounded by tropical greenery. That friendly wave connects the two riders as part of the community of people enjoying their bikes.

This woman was probably on her way to the beach, to work, or to a friend's home. Armstrong was looking for something very different on his morning ride through the green roads of Hawaii. During that season, hours of training rides each day took him up grades approaching 25 percent, or from sea level to 5,000 feet elevation. And yet he's on the road for at least some of the reasons other bikers are: to be outdoors in any kind of weather; to enjoy the sight of new roads and new surroundings; to feel alive and vital, moving at the body's own pace from one place to another. It doesn't matter very much that for Armstrong, the body's own pace is often twice that of the relaxed cyclists he passes.

It's not unusual for bike riders taking long day trips on back roads in their own hometown areas to have the pleasure of finding themselves joining Armstrong on a training ride. Many of these riders report on blogs and in cycling magazines that they were glad to keep up with a world-class athlete for a mile or 10 miles, answering his questions about the roads ahead.

STILL ON THE TEAM

During his second comeback, in May 2009, Armstrong rode in Italy in the Giro d'Italia race. His collarbone was still healing after a bad crash in April. That didn't stop him from getting back to racing and meeting the team Astana schedule. "That's what I'd come to Italy for: to get used to riding with the peloton every day and getting along with the guys."[9]

In the 2009 Giro, the race route followed roads that were familiar to Armstrong from his long history of training rides. One stage took the route outside Italy to Austria, then the next stage led the cyclists back into Italy by way of Switzerland and Saint Moritz. This was an area Armstrong had come to know well between 1999 and 2005. During those years, he usually lived in Saint Moritz for the month of June. These were the roads he trained on before most of his Tour de France wins.

Few professional bike riders are able to spend as much time as Armstrong does training for the major races. Fewer still can afford to live in comfortable conditions instead of a tiny, cheap room with an uncomfortable bed while training. Armstrong finds that riding for many days on the same kinds of roads as the races, and often the actual routes, improves his race performance. So does riding in rough, extreme weather conditions. He also prefers to spend each night of a multistage race in a comfortable hotel or *pension*, with the team's cook preparing pasta and sauce for the evening meal. Usually when staying in these hotels, he has a team member as a roommate.

WORKS WELL WITH OTHERS

Armstrong is not only a team player for his own team, he has also learned to work in solidarity with other cyclists. They are his colleagues as well as his competitors. It may not be fun watching someone else win a race, but he has learned to support his teammates' victories. He can appreciate a rival's good efforts, too.

Over the years, Armstrong has come to feel a strong sense of community within the cycling world. His own leading role in this community was apparent during the Giro in May 2009. Before the ninth stage of the Giro race began, Armstrong met with Dario Cioni, a representative of the Professional Cyclists Association. They were concerned about safety issues for a particularly dangerous stage of the Giro.

"Dangerous" is a relative term for cyclists. After all, these same riders expected that a few days later they would be speeding through Rome on cobblestone roads lined with crowds, with motorcycles and team cars swerving unnervingly close to the peloton. Cyclists are used to assuming some risk during road races.

For this particular stage, the riders would be barreling along at top speed on a road that had train tracks running in their direction of travel. Cars would also be parked in the middle of the road. Their decision was to unite in a boycott of the competition for that day—they would ride the day's route without racing. This decision was supported by a ruling from the UCI: that stage of the race was considered neutralized.

Armstrong recognizes that it's important for a competitive cyclist to work well not only as an individual or a team member, but as one of many riders in a race. Bad manners in an uncooperative rider can lead to unnecessary pressure or even crashes. The riders are packed together and moving at speeds that are hard for even other athletes to comprehend. At the end of a race, cyclists are moving at speeds seen in speed skating, where there are only two competitors on a closed track.

The fourth stage of the 2009 Giro saw Armstrong finish in 32nd place, but only *15 seconds* behind that day's leader. Some three dozen riders finished that day's race at the front of the peloton, packed in five tight groups. With less than half a second between any two riders, there were many chances for collisions that could have caused massive pileups when the rest of the competitors swept in from behind. This illustrates the importance of cooperation, even in the middle of competition.

2009 TOUR DE FRANCE

Armstrong tells a funny story about the team time trial portion of the 2009 Tour de France. For this stage of the race, Armstrong arranged for his friend, actor Ben Stiller, to ride in the team car with Astana's team director, Johan Bruyneel. Stiller came by a few minutes before the team time trial. Seeing video cameras and bikes set up on wind trainers gave Stiller an idea for a funny home video.

Stiller climbed up onto Armstrong's bike on the wind trainer and pretended he was warming up. He cued Armstrong to come for his own warm-up, and when he did, Stiller refused to get off. It was amusing enough for the moment. Then Stiller climbed down off the bike, much less gracefully than Armstrong would have. "He managed to torque the chain so much that it snapped," Armstrong quipped. With about four minutes before the event, this could have been a total disaster. Team mechanics were able to change the chain in time. "The good news is we wound up with a pretty funny video and my new chain held up fine for the stage."[10]

Even with the last-minute chain replacement, Armstrong and the rest of team Astana rode very well during that team time trial. He started that stage of the race some 30 or 40 seconds behind Fabian Cancellara, who was the current leader. No one on the team expected that they would pick up enough time to put Armstrong in the yellow jersey. But they ended up winning the team time trial with a time that was just 22/100ths of a second short of taking the individual lead as well. During interviews held just after the team time trial, Armstrong praised the team's impressive victory. There was no point in complaining about just missing out on wearing the *maillot jaune*. He knew the response to that unhappy thought: ride harder. That's what professional cycling is like for him.

BIGGEST FAN

Lance Armstrong's number one fan is and always has been his mother. But there's a contender for biggest fan. He's certainly bigger in size than tiny Linda Armstrong Kelly.

Though Armstrong doesn't know his name, he recognizes this man at first glance. The fan attended most of the bike races that Armstrong competed in, between 2008 and 2010, cheering from the sidelines. He's big, but there's a lot of muscle in his beefy frame, almost two times as broad as Armstrong's lean five-foot-nine-inch (1.75-meter) figure.

The fan runs alongside part of the race route. At some races, many fans run beside the race leaders where space and crowds permit. It's easy to pick this fan out of the crowd because he alternates between wearing an Armstrong jersey and a helmet with Texas longhorns, and a

Levi Leipheimer jersey and a helmet with elk horns. After a while, he started showing up at the races with a Tyler Farrar jersey and a helmet with eagle wings. Seeing him in costume is a lot of fun for many of the European fans. Armstrong gets a kick out of this costumed fan, as well as others he has seen standing along race routes costumed as angels or devils.

RELATIONS WITH MEDIA

It may seem fun to be the center of attention. Being interviewed has become a normal part of most events that Armstrong does, whether for sports or for the Lance Armstrong Foundation. While he's out doing training rides, he'll get calls from journalists seeking a quick interview or trying to get just one question answered. Most of the time, he handles these calls and informal interviews with the same good grace and good manners he shows during formal television interviews.

Sometimes it's not much fun at all, and not even interesting for him. It's easier for him to enjoy meeting some media people, such as Diane Sawyer, who makes interviews interesting. Some of the journalists who interview Armstrong, such as ESPN's Rick Reilly, have become good friends with him over the years. Not everyone can make an athlete feel comfortable giving an exclusive interview while getting a postrace massage. During the 2009 Tour de France, Reilly was able to ask questions and record answers from Armstrong even while masseur Ryszard Kielpinski was working on the naked athlete's legs and back.

Since Armstrong left professional racing in 2005, public use of Internet social forums like Facebook and Twitter has increased. His second comeback, late in 2008, was promoted with an active presence on the Internet. Thousands of fans receive short messages, or "tweets," that Armstrong types and sends from his cell phone. He's not the only rider who keeps connected with a phone or BlackBerry device, making and receiving phone calls and e-mail.

HOME

Home for Armstrong is any of several places. For him, home might be in the suburbs of Dallas, where he was raised. He bought his mother a fine house in Dallas, and she lives there with her fourth husband.

He has a home in Austin, Texas, where he has lived since he rented his first place of his own. The house he owns now in Austin is only a few minutes away from the home of his ex-wife, Kristin Richards. This allows them to share the parenting of their three children very conveniently when he is in Austin.

Armstrong has a home in Aspen, Colorado, which is convenient for long training rides as well as skiing during the winter. He has owned places in France and in Girona, Spain. These and other similar sites have mostly been a home away from home, an alternative to hotels while he was training far from the United States.

The third home that Armstrong has is a ranch in the Texas hill country, near Dripping Springs. That's where he goes for the peacefulness of wide-open spaces. He looks at the slope of his land and out to the horizon. He rides there, too, skidding on rough gravel roads and dodging pickup trucks on miles of Texas highways.

NOTES

1. Lance Armstrong with Sally Jenkins, *Every Second Counts* (New York: Broadway Books, Random House, 2003), p. 21.

2. Mary Oliver, "The Summer Day," in *New and Selected Poems* (Boston: Beacon Press, 1992).

3. Armstrong, *Every Second Counts*, p. 19.

4. "The Shop," Mellow Johnny's Bike Shop Web site, http://www.mellowjohnnys.com/the-shop.

5. Lance Armstrong, *Comeback 2.0: Up Close and Personal* (New York: Touchstone/Simon and Schuster, 2009), ch. 5.

6. Armstrong, *Comeback 2.0*, ch. 2.

7. Armstrong, *Comeback 2.0*, ch. 2.

8. Armstrong, *Comeback 2.0*, ch. 2.

9. Armstrong, *Comeback 2.0*, ch. 4.

10. Armstrong, *Comeback 2.0*, ch. 4.

Chapter 2

PERSONAL BACKGROUND

Where do champion athletes come from? They have superior bodies, obviously, to perform better at sports than almost anyone else. These bodies come from good genes and good food, combined with good training. But where does the mind of an athlete come from, to guide that superior body through training and performance? The mind is a subtler thing to analyze than the physical body. And in a growing young athlete, the mind is created by a thousand small interactions in life.

It's clear that Lance Armstrong became a champion athlete because he had superior physical abilities. He was born with some of these abilities and did nothing to earn them. "My mother gave me my heart, lungs, arms, legs, and genes. But whatever natural physical abilities I possess were as randomly awarded as the winning numbers on a roulette wheel," Armstrong acknowledged. He knows all too well that being born healthy isn't enough to make someone an athlete or a champion. "Without an organized will and discipline, physical attributes are meaningless. Without the sure-handed parenting I received from Linda Mooneyham Armstrong, they would have amounted to nothing. They'd have been just a collection of scattered characteristics, topped off by a smart mouth."[1]

NATURE VERSUS NURTURE

It's easy to understand that the children of athletes are more likely than average people to do well at sports. However, Armstrong wasn't born to parents who were champion athletes. His birth parents were active in school sports, but not international competitions.

It's also understandable that a parent who is successful at a very demanding career is more likely than most parents to raise children who seek out similar challenges. If so, where did Armstrong's success begin? "How does a supermarket checkout girl produce a son who becomes a Tour de France champion?" asked Armstrong. "The theorists and social psychologists can bicker all they want over the nature versus nurture question, but for me, the matter's settled. It's perfectly clear: I owe it all to my mother. What would I have been without her? A barroom brawler maybe. Or an arsonist."[2]

That statement isn't just empty words. Armstrong has no illusions about the kind of boy and youth he was. He got in scuffles and fights in and out of school. He took more interest in playing with fire than was good for him. As a youth, he had a hot temper. Trash-talking and sports events weren't enough to use up all his drive to compete and win. Without guidance, the odds are good that as a grown man he could have ended up as a hard-drinking Texas roughneck with a fast car and a criminal record.

Instead, he became a world-class athlete and a hero to people around the world. He does have a fast car, too. "I'm many things: a cancer survivor, a father, a Tour de France champion. But I'm one thing before all others, and it's a thing I'm so proud of," wrote Armstrong in the foreword to his mother's autobiography. "I'm a son who seems to have pleased his mother."[3]

TELLING THE STORY

Journalists trying to make good television out of sports coverage often interview Lance Armstrong's mother. She takes their attention in good humor most of the time, knowing that they're looking for the Legend of Mellow Johnny. As she wrote in a memoir of her years growing up and raising young Lance, "They think I somehow made him be the way he is and should be able to tell them how to make their child be that way too, so they can bottle and sell it."[4] She figures that if journalists want to know why her young son loved his bike, perhaps they should ask a little boy. Some people have forgotten the simple truths that balls are for throwing, games are for playing, and bikes are for riding.

Writing a book about your life is an illuminating experience, according to Linda Armstrong Kelly. She thinks that people should be encouraged to write about their own lives. Her son has taken that piece of writing advice more seriously than most people do. With the help of Sally Jenkins and Elizabeth Kreutz, he's written three memoirs of his life, as well as other books about the Lance Armstrong Foundation and his LiveSTRONG program. This is in addition to the many books that *other* people have written *about* him. But the story of Linda Armstrong—born Linda Mooneyham, and now Linda Armstrong Kelly—is also the story of her son, Lance. The story of her success is the story of Lance Armstrong's success.

WHERE IT BEGAN

Lance Armstrong's origins were not the little suburban house with a white picket fence of his mother Linda's fantasies. She had grown up watching a lot of television in the low-rent housing projects of Oak Cliff, a run-down suburb of Dallas, Texas. Her parents were divorced, and young Linda knew what sort of home life she wanted to have one day. There was going to be a beautiful and well-turned-out mother; brothers and sisters playing together; and a confident, hardworking father. Things didn't work out that way for her, starting with an unplanned pregnancy.

Linda Mooneyham may not have planned to become a mother at 17, but once she realized she was expecting, this was not an unwanted pregnancy. She wore her sister Debbie's loose blouses for months, baby-doll tops with gathered bodices and billowy fronts, trying to hide her thickening waist as long as possible. Even the thought of abortion made her feel sick inside, she said years later in her memoir; and in Texas in 1970 there were no options for safe or legal abortions in hospitals. There was no effective sex education in schools at that time, either. The absence of the basic sex education that is common in most North American schools in the 21st century probably contributed to her unplanned pregnancy. But there were lessons that she had learned very thoroughly at home and at school, lessons about consequences and responsibility. She was very sure that her choices had consequences, and she felt responsible for the baby she was expecting.

Her boyfriend, Eddie Gunderson, married Linda on her 17th birthday, almost as soon as they knew she was pregnant. He finished high school and they tried hard to make a life together. On September 18, 1971, their son, Lance Edward Gunderson, was born. Baby Lance weighed nine pounds, 10 ounces at birth. Growing quickly, he kept his parents on their toes, beginning to walk at nine months. But neither of these young parents was ready and able at 17 to make a marriage work. They divorced while their son was still a baby.

MAKING IT WORK

Hard work can make a difference in a person's life, and Armstrong's mother is a testament to the virtues of hard work. Babysitting jobs for

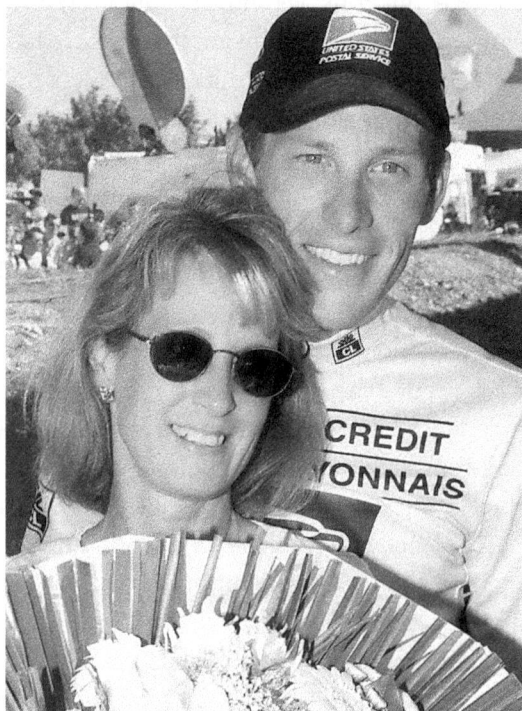

Overall leader Lance Armstrong of the United States poses with his mother, Linda, after winning the 19th stage of the Tour de France cycling race, a 57-kilometer individual time trial around the Futuroscope theme park near Poitiers, France, July 24, 1999. (AP Photo/Michel Spingler)

neighbors were a way to make money for treats and nice things, starting when Linda was only 9 years old. She learned how to save for her goals, and, with the help of her paternal grandmother, how to sew clothes. She worked at Kentucky Fried Chicken before she was 14 to earn the money for her drill team uniform in junior high school. When she was pregnant with Lance, she left high school and worked as a supermarket checkout clerk. She helped her husband, Eddie, deliver newspapers at night. When Lance was a baby, she worked at the U.S. Post Office for the Christmas rush and in the dead-letter department.

While Lance was still small, Linda got her GED high school equivalency, but she wasn't able to go on to college or university. The lack of higher education limited the kinds of jobs she was able to find. For years she worked at two jobs and sometimes three. She could rely on her family and Eddie's mother to babysit Lance during the hours not covered by preschool. This work wasn't just for money. It was for focusing her energies on making her life better, as she had in school through the teamwork and positive attitude of the drill team. Now she was focused on making a home for her family and being the parent her boy needed.

Every setback was an opportunity to achieve something else in a different way. She made it her business to find the opportunity in every setback and to apply the necessary hard work to give that opportunity a chance for success. Obstacles were not failures, they were something to overcome.

It's clear not only to Armstrong, looking back at his mother's early adult years, but to anyone who knows single parents that his mother must have been exhausted much of the time and even desperate on occasion. As a child and a youth, he respected how hard she worked to make a home for him. He remembers her as always cheerful and full of energy, as always having time to read to him every evening when he was little. By the age of two, he was reciting the books' verses with her, learning to read. She remembers playing with him, rough-and-tumble games and board games with dice, trying to tire out her high-energy child so he would fall asleep.

She got up early every morning to make him a hot breakfast, usually biscuits and gravy but sometimes eggs and bacon or waffles for special occasions. She would tidy their home every morning, before he went

to day care or school and she went to work. They ate dinner by candle-
light, and she insisted on good table manners. Even Hamburger Helper
or macaroni and cheese is not just food, it's dinner to Linda; it's the
time when a family sits down together, lights candles, and talks nicely
about their day. Since they got up early together, they went to sleep
early as well.

Armstrong doesn't remember her ever complaining about being
tired or having too much to do. As a grown man and father, he has
come to understand just how much hard work and positive attitude she
put into each day of his youth. Her refusal to acknowledge limits—for
herself or for him—shaped him as a boy. "We were partners in carving
out better lives for ourselves," he said in her memoir, "and we fought for
each other, back to back against our obstacles."[5]

When young Lance told her there was a running race at school he
was going to enter, Linda praised him. She gave him a good-luck piece
to carry in his sock when he ran. It was a silver dollar that she'd gotten in her change and hung onto, because it was minted the year that
her son was born. She suggested that if he put his mind to it, he could
become an athlete and compete at the Olympics. He won that running
race. He carried that good-luck piece for years at races. And he never
forgot that his mother believed he could be an Olympian if he really
put his mind to it.

A STEPFATHER FOR LANCE

With Linda's childhood dreams of having a home and family like those
she saw on television sitcoms, it's no surprise that she was willing to
marry a second time. When her son Lance was three years old, she married Terry Armstrong. It takes a special kind of man to marry a woman
who already has a child. For a while Linda thought Terry Armstrong
was the man for her.

It seems Terry thought so, too. Both he and Linda worked, and with
their combined incomes it was possible to live in a nice neighborhood.
Terry legally adopted Lance and gave him his name. His own parents
didn't get on as well with Lance or Linda. Linda felt that perhaps they
were disappointed that their son had no other children with Linda
other than the son he had adopted and given his name.

Terry Armstrong was the adopted son of a minister. He tried to impose his religious values on his stepson, but he had a temper as well. His idea of discipline included spanking with a wooden paddle from his fraternity days. There were spankings for being messy, for coming home late, and for making smart-aleck comments. This kind of discipline didn't encourage a warm father-son relationship. It was also one of the things that made young Lance decide that his stepfather was a hypocrite. Lance decided to have nothing to do with that kind of religion.

While Lance's mother worked hard to make their family life as much like the television fantasies as she could, Lance's stepfather was a traveling salesman. Terry Armstrong traveled a lot for business; he was on the road most of the time and usually home only on weekends. As the years went by he seemed less involved with Linda and Lance. He did bring home a dog for the family, though. It was a white spitz that shed hair everywhere and slept on Lance's bed.

PROGRESS

The family's progress could be tracked on a map of the Dallas area as they moved through a succession of increasingly better neighborhoods. Their first apartment was a one-bedroom in Oak Cliff, a run-down neighborhood in Dallas. They moved to a rental house in Garland, a nearby suburb, where Lance joined the YMCA football and soccer teams. Terry coached the football team for two years. With a good job as a secretary, Linda was able to get a nicer apartment in nearby Richardson, Texas. There Lance was signed up for swimming lessons. He was also given his first good bicycle.

The swimming lessons were for the City of Plano Swimmers, at the country club in nearby Plano. The Armstrongs weren't the country-club type, but the pool was close enough to their home that Lance could ride there on his bike. Lance's school friends had been swimming for a couple of years already. After starting with the beginners, Lance managed to catch up to his middle-school age group in a month. He caught the coach's attention. A year later, at the state competition he took fourth in the 1,500-meter freestyle.

In Plano, another suburb of Dallas, Lance's mother got her best job yet, as a secretary with a telecommunications company. The family was able to buy a home. It was a good neighborhood, a few blocks from Dooley Elementary School. Within three miles were the schools that Lance attended over the next several years: Armstrong Middle School, Williams High, and Plano East High. Over the next several years Linda worked her way up in the telecommunications company. Eventually she became an account manager. The job included training newly hired people much younger than she was, with bachelor's degrees from colleges and universities.

Without a degree, it seemed there was only so far Linda could advance at work. She began to plan for the future, when Lance would be in high school. Maybe he would get a sports scholarship and go on to college to study engineering or computer science. By the time Lance was 15, his mother was able to go to night school and take some business courses. She even realized one of her dreams and got her real estate license. It was wonderful to sell houses, even if much of the extra money she made went toward the costs of getting Lance to the sports events he enjoyed so much; new sports gear, entry fees, and the costs of travel.

This giving didn't go in only one direction. After one of his triathlon victories, Linda got to hear her teenaged son say on television that he was so excited to win. Sometimes he even won a cash prize, he told the interviewer from *KidSports* on ESPN, and that really helped his mom, who didn't have a lot of money. She never forgot that moment, one of the first television interviews in a life that was later to become crowded with media attention. Even in the middle of the exciting buzz he felt after winning a triathlon, young Lance remembered his mom. He knew that it took money to make his home and his exciting sports activities happen. He understood that his mother worked hard for what she gave him.

FIRST BICYCLES

The first bike Lance rode was a little tricycle of the "Big Wheel" or "Green Machine" style. It was a present from his mother for his second birthday. It didn't take long for him to figure out how to make it go. Like many toddlers, he seemed to want to go everywhere at once. And when he realized that pedaling faster made the bike move faster, he was off and scooting around as fast as he could go.

For Christmas when he was still small, Lance was given a little bike. His grandfather put air in the tires and tuned it up. And Lance was off, weaving around kids on skateboards and the neighborhood dogs.

For his seventh birthday, Lance's mother and stepfather got him his first really good bike, a BMX racing bike from Richardson Bike Mart. Linda knew that being at day care until she finished work for the day was hard on her boy, so she tried to help him use up as much of his excess energy as possible when they got home. The newspaper had run an article one day about bicycle motocross racing in the Dallas area. BMX racing sounded like an interesting sport, and there were events for boys as young as kindergarten age. Jim Hoyt, the bike store owner, had noticed Lance and his mother going by the bike store every weekend. He gave her a good deal on a brown Schwinn Mag Scrambler with yellow mag wheels. The BMX bike and safety gear cost three times more than Linda had hoped to spend on a gently used bike. She learned quickly that there are no "gently used" BMX bicycles, not after they've been ridden on the rough courses.

The expense of that new bike for such a young child caused some financial stress. But like Linda, Terry Armstrong saw the good sense in getting the child active in outdoor sports for good health. Baseball was another good sport he knew, so he coached Lance's Little League team and got him a good catcher's mitt. As the football coach, Terry was pleased with their team's performance. The Armstrong family did some activities like this together, but as Lance grew older, most of the time it was his mother who took him to weekend sports events and cheered him on.

A GOOD ROAD BIKE

Lance's first good road bike was a Mercier, slim and elegant, bought when he was 13. While hanging around the Richardson Bike Mart, Lance saw a flyer for the IronKids junior triathlon. It was the first time he'd ever heard of a triathlon, but he was good at biking, swimming, and running. It didn't take any convincing to get his mother to agree to let him sign up for the event. He needed a triathlon outfit with a fast-drying shirt and cross-training shorts so he could go from one phase of the event to the next without changing clothes. He also needed a good racing bike, so that's why the Mercier was bought.

Bikes may seem like an indulgence or a luxury at first glance. It's not every parent who buys a young child good bicycles and gear, first for BMX racing and then for road racing. But Linda was keeping track. She wrote later in her memoir that she felt it was better to have her boy active in sports than to find him sitting at home on the couch eating potato chips every day when she came home from work. By age 13, Lance was riding to swim practice before school, at times riding to school, and then riding to swim practice again after classes. Any activity that could keep her high-energy boy out of trouble was something she wanted to encourage. A bicycle for Lance was not just a toy left rusting in the yard. It was transportation while his mother was busy at work. This was a way he could do the sports he enjoyed and stay out of trouble.

FIRST BICYCLE INJURY

The first bicycle injury Lance Armstrong ever had came long before his BMX days and not long after the plastic tricycle. He was still a small boy, and he fell off an adult bicycle when he was riding with his birth father.

For a while after his parents divorced, Lance would spend Saturday afternoons with his father and grandmother, Willene Gunderson. One day, he went for his first bicycle ride with his father and took a tumble. Maybe he wasn't hanging on as tightly as the adults thought. They took him right to the hospital for a couple of stitches. They called his mother to let her know he would be fine, staying at his grandmother's home that night. But she was panicked by the news and frantic when they didn't bring him home till the next morning. This was part of the reason that shared parenting didn't work for them.

There was no lasting physical injury for Lance, though. For him, this was the first in a series of bike-related injuries, mostly small cuts and bruises and road rashes from falls. When he started swimming lessons and triathlon training, it seemed as though he always had small injuries like these that would take a while to heal because of the pool water. His mother used to joke that they should have bought stock in Spenco

2nd Skin. This lightweight, clear bandage was the best dressing for his scrapes.

AN ACTIVE BOY

It was always easy to find young Lance playing outside. He made his own sound effects and chanted his own theme music. Often he played at being Steve Austin, hero of the television show *The Six Million Dollar Man*. "We can rebuild him!" he'd chant, leaping over hedges. "Better . . . stronger . . . faster!" Still, it took more than just letting Lance run around a park or open field to wear him out by the end of a day.

Sports weren't all the same to this growing boy. He tried Little League, but hand-eye coordination was not his strong point. Neither was football, and this could have been a real disappointment. A Texas boy no good at football? Football was the sport that mattered the most in middle school and later at Plano East High School. But any ball sports, especially if they involved moving from side to side, needed a kind of coordination that Lance just didn't have. He didn't like that in team sports, one person's slip could affect the whole team's score.

He did show coordination while running, though, and on his bike. Neighbors would complain to his mother that Lance had been leaping over their hedges. Drivers had to hit the brakes abruptly when he came riding down the street. Lance also showed a knack for getting in scuffles with other boys. It seemed for a while that every teacher or neighbor and even the swim coach brought complaints to Linda. Teachers said that he was bright and would do well in school if he applied himself. Linda thought he was applying himself pretty well to many things. One of them was learning. He had a dictionary on his desk at home. For years, he would learn a new word every day. He did his homework and was busy in a variety of activities.

Far from being a micromanaging parent, Linda was a working mother who had to trust that her latchkey kid wouldn't burn down the house after school. Those are not just empty words that most working parents might say about their kids. She didn't know that 12-year-old Lance and his buddy Steve Lewis had invented a game. They would put gasoline in a plastic dishpan and float tennis balls in it. Then they would pick out a ball and light it with a match, setting it aflame. Lance and Steve played catch with the flaming balls many times, wearing oven mitts or garden gloves. Many disasters were narrowly avoided, with Lance on occasion having to climb onto the roof to stamp out shingles that caught fire. Still, the house never burned down, even when the dishpan of gasoline caught fire and melted down into the yard.

WHAT WAS NEVER SAID

Looking back on his years growing up, Armstrong doesn't complain about the absence of his birth father or the feeling that his stepfather had become less active in his daily life. Instead, he's amazed that his young mother somehow managed to fill the roles of two parents— breadwinner and homemaker—at once. He grew up feeling that he had everything that he needed or wanted, and he knew how to reach his goals. So many times she told him to make an opportunity out of every setback. But he realizes now that there were so many other things that a parent could easily say that she never said to him.

So many parents might end up saying at the end of a long, tiring day, "Get off your bike and come indoors." It would be easy after paying for yet another BMX event for a parent to snarl about being fed up with the expense of replacing equipment again and again. Parents could be frustrated by kids trying to win state and regional competitions against older and better-trained competitors. It's understandable that some parents might tell their kids not to be too ambitious; it might be better to settle for less than being the best. Don't pin your hopes too high, is something parents might say to spare their children the disappointment of not being the absolute best. A hardworking parent trying to stretch the family budget could suggest that working at a local grocery or department store might be a better pastime for a teenager than going to sports events and competitions. But Linda Armstrong never said any of these things to her son.

Day by day, she gave him the benefits of her work ethic and attitude. She tried to help her son make the most of the gifts of his healthy, strong body. He grew up to be an Olympian. He became a world-class athlete in one of the most challenging sports in the world.

Armstrong didn't properly understand how hard it is to be a parent until he became a father himself. "It seems to me that rearing a child is the trickiest job in the world," he said in his mother's memoir. "Every word and gesture can have unintended consequences, and a large mistake can mean the difference between a whole, healthy, self-fulfilled human being and a deprived and self-defeating one."[6]

WHO'S YOUR DADDY?

It may be hard for some people to understand, but Lance Armstrong and his mother have never talked about his father. Not even when he might have been dying of cancer, not even when he had children of his own. Never.

Who is Lance Armstrong's real father—the man who sired him, or the man who adopted him and gave him his name? If a "real" father is a man who is there over and over for a child, doing supportive things, perhaps Lance's grandfather Paul Mooneyham qualifies. Becoming a grandfather was a pivotal moment in Mooneyham's life. When Lance was born, Mooneyham joined Alcoholics Anonymous and got his life in order. He was particularly supportive during the first years of Lance's life, when it was hardest for his young mother to make a home. When Lance was emerging as a young triathlete, his grandfather made a particular point of attending triathlon events. At the Waco, Texas, events, Mooneyham would wear a shirt that read in bold letters: "I'm Lance's Papa!"

Lance's birth father did try to live up to his responsibilities. Eddie Gunderson married Lance's mother and tried to make it work. After their divorce she was angry with him for years. Eventually she came to understand that Gunderson wasn't ready for marriage and fatherhood at that time. Armstrong wrote in his memoir *Every Second Counts* that his father might as well have been "an anonymous DNA donor" because he left when Lance was so young. Surrendering all legal parental rights to his son looks like abandonment, especially when Gunderson signed papers a few years later permitting Linda's second husband to adopt Lance. But it can also be seen as a way to show respect for her new marriage, and for Linda's ability to care for their son. It's possible this surrender was a way of not interfering, of not imposing himself in her life with her new husband. Being absent may have been a way he was able to show consideration for them, instead of being present and making wrong choices that the new family would resent.

A story in Linda Armstrong's memoir tells of the dark days when her grown son was at his sickest during his cancer treatments. Her father came to sit with her in a hospital waiting room and confided that Eddie Gunderson had come up to him at a store that week. Gunderson had taken the opportunity to catch up with his former father-in-law, talking about his new family and asking about Lance. Gunderson had seen on television that Lance was being treated for cancer. He wanted to come by the hospital and see Lance, perhaps because he thought Lance might be dying. The reaction from Linda was to tell her father a flat *no*. She didn't want anyone to burden her son's mind with any other concerns at this time. And she believed there was no way her son was going to die from this cancer.

A few years later, Armstrong read in a newspaper article that his birth father once tried to contact him after he won the 1999 Tour de France. Armstrong had no interest in knowing the man or dwelling on him, and made no welcome for him among the people handling his business contacts. "He was the keeper of the secret, the man with the answer to the unanswerable," wrote Armstrong in *Every Second Counts*. "I intended to investigate the meanings of family through my own children—by looking ahead, not back."[7]

FINDING FATHERS

Sometimes father figures are people who come into a young person's life and behave as a father should behave. Father figures help by teaching, guiding, and holding the young person accountable to a standard of behavior. Uncles are certainly people on whom growing children depend. Lance's uncle, Alan Mooneyham, was a reliable babysitter while Linda was working. He was there at family gatherings. Sometimes he and other family members attended Lance's sport events, cheering with Linda.

Lance's swimming coach from Plano, Chris MacCurdy, was one of the sporting people who took a lasting interest in Lance. He trained Lance as a swimmer from middle school through high school, encouraging him to consider competing nationally and training for the Olympics. He felt that Lance could earn a full scholarship to a good college.

The owner of the Bike Mart in Richardson took a lasting interest in Lance. Jim Hoyt started by giving the boy's mother good prices on better equipment than she could afford. In high school, Lance had the equivalent of a part-time job riding for events sponsored by Hoyt's store.

When Lance first moved out to live on his own, he rented a small home in Austin from J. T. Neal. This supporter of emerging athletes kept an eye on Lance over the years as his life kept changing.

In some ways, Armstrong has never really missed having a father in his life. There are men who serve a fatherly role for him in many ways. One was Jim Ochowicz, the team manager who signed Armstrong to a professional cycling team sponsored by Motorola. Not only did he direct the young cyclist in becoming a seasoned professional, he taught him about life—good food, getting along with people—while traveling with the team.

Another father substitute is Eddy Merckx, the man Armstrong considers the finest cyclist ever. "The same July a man first set foot on the moon, Merckx won the first of his five Tours de France," editor Loren Mooney said of him in *Bicycling* magazine. "In his career he would win five Giros d'Italia, one Vuelta a España, three world championships, three Paris-Roubaix and more than two dozen other Spring Classics. . . . He is universally admired, and for good reason. Merckx still epitomizes grace on the bike."[8] He has taken a lasting interest in Armstrong's career choices, and his good advice was a welcome support during Armstrong's second comeback in 2009.

SAYING THANKS—AND MEANING IT

The words "thank you" can be easy to say. That simple phrase can be ordinary and everyday. Used over and over, it can be a sign of many small kindnesses over a lifetime. But how do you properly thank a parent who has clearly done more than mere duty?

As a youth, Armstrong tried to show his appreciation for his mom's dedication and hard work. As a man, he tried to express adequately his gratitude for her gifts—not only her work to house and support him, but her good attitude and her delight in his strength and joy. In many ways, he tried over the years to thank her properly, with words and presents.

Armstrong did come close to succeeding once, as he awoke after brain surgery with the fog of anesthetic still clouding his mind. He asked the nurses for his mother, and she was at his bedside in moments.

"I want you to know how much I love my life," he told her, "and how much I love you for giving it to me."[9]

NOTES

1. Lance Armstrong, foreword to *No Mountain High Enough: Raising Lance, Raising Me*, by Linda Armstrong Kelly with Joni Rodgers (Waterville, ME: Thorndike Press, 2005), p. 13.

2. Ibid.

3. Ibid., p. 18.

4. Kelly, *No Mountain High Enough*, p. 28.

5. Armstrong, foreword, *No Mountain High Enough*, p. 16.

6. Ibid., p. 14.

7. Lance Armstrong with Sally Jenkins, *Every Second Counts* (New York: Broadway Books, Random House, 2003), p. 28.

8. Loren Mooney, "86 Miles With Eddy Merckx," *Bicycling*, October 2009, p. 10.

9. Armstrong, foreword, *No Mountain High Enough*, p. 18.

Chapter 3

STARTING OUT

As a teenager, Lance Armstrong began serious training as an athlete. At the age of 14, Lance won a duathlon (swimming and running) at an upscale health club in Dallas. The prize was a $100 pair of Avia running shoes! But the pair that arrived in the mail didn't fit. The local sales representative, Scott Eder, came over to make good on the prize. The young man ended up becoming a sports mentor to Lance. With Linda Armstrong's approval, Eder took her son and his friends on workouts and to events. Eder made sure that Lance was welcome again at the Richardson Bike Mart, after some bad-tempered behavior had gotten him thrown out.

Fireworks and water balloons were pranks Lance and his friends used to enjoy. They also figured out how to sneak bottles of beer out of fridges in neighbor's garages and run away with them down the alley. At age 15, he and a friend argued with a neighbor and glued the man's mailbox shut. The police took an interest in that incident, and in the "Armstrong Street" sign that he'd taken for his room.

GETTING ORGANIZED

As Lance began high school, his mother noticed positive changes in his behavior. "He stayed out of the kind of trouble that had always seemed to find him during middle school," Linda Armstrong wrote in her memoir. That was very welcome, as she had decided to divorce her husband, Terry. When she told her son of the divorce, she asked him not to get into any trouble. She just wasn't able to handle it at that time. Lance came through for her. No problems at school, and he tried not to fight with other boys. "With all his energy in demand at every event, he stopped channeling so much of it toward getting angry at people,"[1] she noticed. They spent most weekends together, driving to 10K runs and triathlons where Lance competed. They were a team.

Trying hard not to make trouble, Lance tried to keep busy at sports with his friends Adam Wilk, Chann Rae, and John Boggan. They went riding, past Southfork (a ranch that appeared on the TV series *Dallas*), and in summer they'd go around Lake Lavon. He even hung the Christmas lights along the roof of the house. Of course, he took the opportunity to moon a few passing cars as well.

Since triathlons and bike races meant so much to her son, Linda encouraged him to find ways to make it possible to attend more events. She gave him a Rolodex to keep track of possible sponsors. Sometimes he was given jerseys, or even shoes. Every sponsor, large or small, got a handwritten letter of thanks from Lance. His mother proudly sewed the sponsors' logos onto his jersey.

Competitive cycling has four categories of riders. Category 1 is the highest level. Lance started out in Category 4 on Tuesday night criterion rides at the Bike Mart. These "Cat 4" races at the Tuesday Crits kept him busy for a while. Then he convinced the organizers to let him ride in a Cat 3 race. They agreed, just to give him some experience. When he won, they upgraded him. By the age of 16, Lance began training with a couple of Cat 1 riders who were local heroes in their late twenties.

"In the evenings I would train for my budding career as a triathlete, and sometimes I would ask her to drive behind me as I rode my bike, to check my times and count the miles. She would grab her car keys, and off we would go," Armstrong remembered for the foreword to his mother's memoir. In those days, his bike didn't have a gadget to keep track of his speed or distance traveled. "She never said, 'I'm too tired.' And she taught me to never say it either."[2]

Those evenings spent together were good times. Linda's car had a music player. With the passenger windows open, Lance could enjoy the music as he rode beside his mom's car. He would always pick music by Metallica or other heavy metal bands. He'd call out to his mother to turn the music louder.

Metallica was often the music he played at home, too. Once in a while Lance would realize that his mother was coming home after a hard day at work. He'd turn off the Guns n' Roses or other heavy metal music. Just for her he'd put on some Kenny G or mellow country music.

"Conscious of our tight finances, he worked his Rolodex to get sponsors for every event and was thrilled when he won any amount of money, large or small," his mother was proud to say. Every event he attended improved his rank, until he was the state champion. "He no longer had to pay an entry fee for certain events. And he was adamant about not paying when he didn't have to."[3]

ROAD RAGE

Lance's beautiful Mercier road racing bike didn't last as long as it should have. He was riding his bike along a country road near Dallas when a truck driver ran him off the road. It sure felt deliberate, so while lying there on the side of the road, Lance flashed a rude hand gesture at the driver. He used a couple of the words he'd picked up when his mom wasn't around.

The truck driver pulled over and got out in a rage. Lance had to run, ducking a gas can the driver threw at him. He saw his bike get stomped. He also saw the number on the truck's license plate and reported it to the police.

Charges were filed. Lance's mother took the truck driver to court and won. Her insurance covered the loss of the bike, allowing Linda to buy her son a Raleigh with racing wheels.

TO SHAVE OR NOT TO SHAVE?

As a boy Armstrong learned that pushing himself to ride his bike fast and for long distances meant that he had to expect a few falls. As a competitive rider, he learned the hard way that going faster and farther meant that he suffered more than just a few bruises and scrapes. He lost track of how many times he tired himself out riding most of the way to Oklahoma and back. After a fall, he was often sore and scraped, with road rash from rough pavement, gravel embedded in his skin, or deep cuts. He learned to pick out the grit and gravel, scrub away the dirt, clean his wounds properly, and cover his wounds with a light dressing.

How can you tell a real cyclist from someone just out for a day's ride on a bike? One way is to look at the cyclist's legs. Don't look for the muscles under the skin. Look at the skin, to see if the cyclist shaves off the hair.

Cyclists aren't the only athletes who shave. Some swimmers shave their entire bodies. Armstrong was a competitive swimmer in his early teens, and he noticed that some swimmers shaved before a major event. Swimmers do this to streamline their bodies, helping them to move smoothly through the water. Shaving might improve the body's speed and aerodynamic efficiency.

Cyclists shave their legs, and sometimes their arms too, but for a different reason. Shaving might streamline their bodies a little, but it doesn't increase their speed through the air by much. Air isn't as thick as water, after all. The most dedicated cyclists, professional and amateur, spend a lot of time on their bikes. They know that they will get cuts and scrapes and even worse injuries. It's a lot easier to clean out the wounds if their skin is shaved smooth. Armstrong learned this the hard way, from doing first aid after his own falls. It's also a lot easier to remove bandages from smooth skin than it is to pull medical tape off a hairy leg or arm.

BOUNCING BACK

That beautiful Raleigh racing bike bought with insurance money didn't end up lasting for long. Lance was hit by a large SUV when he was running yellow lights, and the bicycle was smashed. He was thrown over the bike's handlebars and then across the hood of the SUV, landing on the pavement headfirst and rolling to the curb. Given that he wasn't wearing a helmet, it was a miracle that his injuries were as simple as a twisted knee, cuts in his foot and on his head, and a concussion. The emergency room staff were amazed that he hadn't been killed or paralyzed.

There was a triathlon in six days in Louisville, Lance told the doctor treating him. The doctor told him to go home and do nothing for three weeks: don't walk, don't run, just rest that twisted knee in its heavy brace. So Lance tried to lie around and heal.

He got bored after a couple of days and went to a little local golf course to play a round. It felt better to be up and moving around, so he took off the knee brace. After cutting the stitches in his foot with a nail clipper, he cut holes in his expensive running shoe and bike shoe so his healing foot wouldn't rub.

At the triathlon, he was first out of the water of Dallas Lake. He was first off the bike he had borrowed from a friend. At the end of the 10K run, he was third overall. The Dallas newspaper carried a big article the next day, about how Lance had finished third, six days after being hit by a car. The doctor who treated him in the emergency room couldn't believe it.

The powerful muscles of Lance's neck and shoulders had saved his neck from being broken. Years of swimming and doing laps during training and practices had prepared him for competitions. All that swimming also protected him at a vulnerable moment, although a helmet would have helped protect his head and might have saved him from a concussion. Lance was a triathlete and a competitive cyclist by his high school years, not strictly a swimmer. Even so, the physical results of years of swimming laps every day were long-lasting as he continued to exercise and train.

His classic swimmer's build didn't really change for years. Changing his workouts from swimming to mostly riding didn't change the shape of his body as much as he expected. It took surviving cancer and chemotherapy in his twenties to change the shoulder-heavy proportion of his body to the slimmer balance of a competitive cyclist.

JUNIOR AND SENIOR

High school wasn't the be-all and end-all of young Lance Armstrong's life. He had friends and dates among the popular kids. There were social pressures in Plano to buy fancy consumer goods, to "keep up with the Joneses." As much as he could, Lance ignored those pressures. It took all his mom could earn to keep their family in their nice home. His clothes were clean and ironed but not expensive. Some of the popular kids said he ought to be embarrassed to wear Lycra bike shorts. Lance figured that they should be embarrassed to wear Polo shirts and other designer-label clothing like a uniform. He went to class, but the high school scene wasn't the center of his attention.

Some of his school friends were trying pot or other drugs, but Lance didn't get into that. For one thing, he had enough thrills at competitions. For another, he was often asleep by 9 or 10 at night, worn out from swimming practices and riding his bike. He had another circle of friends as well, in school and outside it—bike racers and runners, some of them professional adult triathletes.

He traveled to Colorado, New Mexico, and other states. During his junior year, he got a passport so that he could compete at a triathlon in the Caribbean with Scott Eder. The summer after grade 11, Lance and John Boggan stayed with a friend of Scott Eder's in San Diego. They slept on couches after long days swimming, biking in the southern California hills, and running with many of the top professional triathletes.

A cartoon posted at xkcd.com shows a graph of 11th-grade activities and rates their usefulness to career success. There's a small bar on the graph for 900 hours of classes, and a smaller bar for 400 hours of homework. But "one weekend messing with PERL" (a computer programming language) has a huge bar. The caption notes, "And the 10 minutes striking up a conversation with that strange kid in home room sometimes matters more than every other part of high school combined."[4] The cartoon was made by a computer enthusiast, of course. If a version of this cartoon were made for Lance's grade 11 activities, instead of messing with a computer language, that weekend activity would be racing at a bike event. The 10-minute conversation would probably be with Scott Eder, or an adult triathlete who called Lance "junior," or maybe with Jim Hoyt at his Bike Mart in Richardson.

Going to class and doing homework were useful for career success, because they were practice in how to learn and keep track of information. These were useful life skills as well. Armstrong used these skills as an emerging professional cyclist racing in Europe, learning languages and how to get along in new places. Later, at age 25, when his cancer was diagnosed, these were skills that Armstrong needed and used to learn everything he could about cancer. While he was in high school, spending most weekends on his bike helped Lance be sure what career he wanted.

BEHIND THE WHEEL

In high school, Lance got a learner's permit and learned to drive. He drove fast whenever he could, in a little red Fiat Spider convertible. One Christmas season he got a part-time job, working night shifts at a Toys R Us. After work, he would drag race with his friend Steve Lewis on the way home through dark streets. Getting a driver's license didn't stop him from such tricks.

Driving fast meant that Lance got ticketed by the police for speeding. Again and again, his mother paid the speeding fines. Somehow, she managed to keep her insurance for her own car and the Fiat. This was one problem with her boy that never seemed to get better, no matter what she said to him.

Lance liked fast cars so much, he bought a Camaro. On paper, Jim Hoyt owned the Camaro, because he helped Lance by signing for the bank loan. Lance drove the Camaro and kept it at home. He covered all the payments—about $5,000 worth—and insurance with money he earned racing for Hoyt's team as well as prizes from races.

UNUSUAL METABOLISM

The prestigious Cooper Clinic in Dallas, the place where the aerobic exercise revolution began, invited Scott Eder to bring 16-year-old Lance Armstrong in for some testing. The clinic's lab researchers know how bodies use oxygen during exercise. A person's VO_2 max is a way to calculate how much oxygen that person takes in and uses. A couch potato might use only 45 or 50 percent of the oxygen in each breath, while athletes often score in the 60s. According to the Cooper Clinic's tests, Lance had the highest VO_2 max that they had ever seen—79.5 percent. Twelve years later, no one had scored higher.

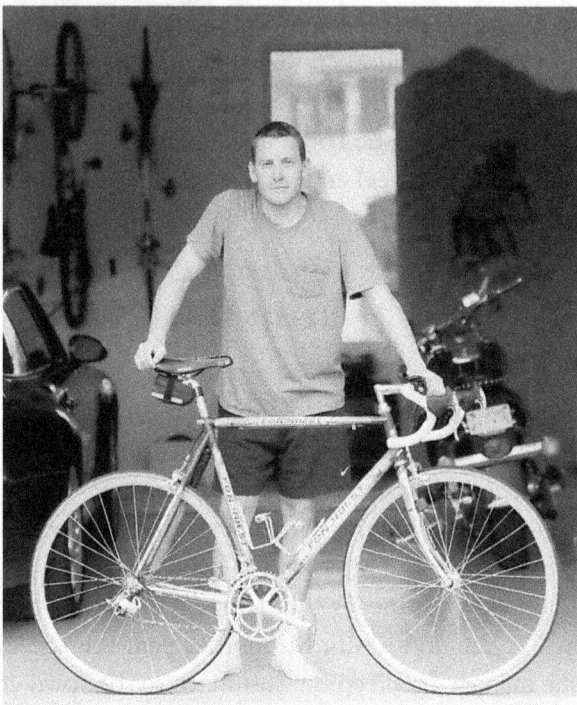

Lance Armstrong in his garage at his home in Austin, Texas, on March 17, 1997. (AP Photo/Harry Cabluck)

Other tests at the Cooper Clinic showed that he produced less lactic acid during exercise than most people. Lactic acid is produced by hard-working muscles and is what causes a person's legs to ache when running for a long time. At 16, Lance had the highest lactic acid threshold they had ever measured.

The tests made it official: he was a natural athlete. He breathed more efficiently than anyone else. He hurt less after hard work than most people. He responded to regular exercise by becoming even more physically fit than before. It was no wonder he was starting to get attention from sports media and sponsors. Yet, even with his natural gifts, there were things he had to learn about using his body well.

EATING RIGHT

Lance made a mistake before one of the first professional triathlons he entered. He ate badly. Eating a couple of cinnamon rolls washed down with two colas doesn't sound like a bad decision. It sounds like an ordinary lunch or snack for a growing boy living in a modern city. Many teenagers in the midst of a growth spurt would eat that and walk around for the rest of the afternoon without a second thought.

But a triathlon isn't an ordinary afternoon spent walking around. After swimming hard and being first out of the water, Lance rode hard and was first off his bike. He began the running part of the race at the front of the pack. He couldn't hold that position. He bonked, which is what riders and runners call the feeling of completely running out of energy and being unable to go on.

So many people passed him that his mother, watching from the finish line, became concerned. Linda walked out for miles along the race course until she found him, limping and exhausted. He was ready to collapse and wanted to quit. She walked beside her son and told him never to quit, whatever he did. He might have to walk, but he would finish. They walked the rest of the way together.

Bonking was a terrible experience. It wasn't the last time he bonked, but he paid attention to the feeling. For subsequent competitions, he tried to eat nutritious food that would give him a steady supply of fuel in his blood sugar.

Instead of cheap white-bread cinnamon rolls from a store, the usual snack that Lance ate was his mother's homemade banana bread. Her recipe made a nutritious and tasty loaf heavy enough to get him through many a day of long rides to pools or lakes for swimming practice, or nighttime rides in endurance races. Years later, Linda still makes banana bread for her grandchildren, and they love it as much as her boy did.

WARM-UP GEAR

There was a time trial in Moriarty, New Mexico, a 12-mile (about 19-km) race for young riders. Lance signed up to ride it in September 1988 during his senior year in high school. Linda drove him to the event, but he packed his own gear.

At six o'clock on the morning of the race, he left their little motel room wearing only a short-sleeved jersey and bike shorts. Linda was getting ready for the day a little more slowly. When they got a motel room for any of these events, they had to save money. The room was always cheap and small with a single bed, and she would sleep on the floor. After only five minutes on his warm-up ride, Lance came back. In that mountain air, he was too cold to ride. But he had forgotten to bring a jacket.

The only warm clothing either of them had was his mother's little pink windbreaker. He wore it. The sleeves didn't come any farther than his elbows, and it barely zipped around him. He wore it all through his warm-up ride. At the starting area, he kept it on and asked Linda to start her car and turn the heater on full blast. Huddling in front of the heat vents, he tried to stay warm until it was his turn to start.

Then he got out of the car, peeled out of the little windbreaker, and got onto his bike. He beat the course record by 45 seconds that day. And, as his mother was pleased to note, he never again forgot to pack a jacket in his gear.

Remembering his gear had always been his own responsibility. Starting back when he was in middle school and going to his first swim meets, it was up to him to pack his own gear bag. If he forgot his swim goggles, Linda didn't run to the sporting goods store and buy him a new pair. She didn't have money for that. She believed that Lance would pay more attention to his preparations if he faced the consequences of forgetting something he needed. She remembered also that when her son was little, he always wanted to carry his own lunch to day care.

GRADUATING CLASS OF '89

The school administrators at Plano East High School objected to how much time Lance spent traveling. He was often away competing, first at triathlons and then at bike events, instead of attending school. His teachers saw these absences as losing focus on the importance of school. They wrote on his report cards that Lance could get better grades if he would just stay focused.

There was plenty of focus in Lance's life, though, according to his mother and coaches. He was focused on his bike and the skills he would need as a world-class athlete. He had a Rolodex full of sponsors, and after each event he wrote to thank each one for their support, even if it was as simple as a free shirt. There was a stack of trophies and ribbons that he'd won. During his senior year, the issue came to a final showdown.

It seemed the school administrators regarded his time away from classes as unexcused absences. They treated his absences as if he was playing hooky to hang out at the mall. In his senior year, they told Lance that he shouldn't travel to Colorado to train with the national team and then go to Moscow to compete in the Junior World Championships.

It seems an odd thing for the school administrators to tell a student who was ranked nationally at the top of his sport. Couldn't they be flexible about worthwhile activities? Another member of that senior class had no problem getting permission to attend the World Junior competition in swimming, but that student wasn't seen as a trouble-maker.

Unfortunately, cycling wasn't a sport recognized by Texas high schools at that time. Football was something the administrators might have understood. After all, there were college scholarship programs for football players. But bike athletes competed in an odd, quirky sport. These guys shaved their legs! There were no crowded stadiums full of cheering bike fans in Texas. And certainly the administrators running Plano East High School when Lance came back from training and competing in the Junior World Championships were not his fans.

Six weeks before graduation, Lance had already bought his prom ticket and paid for his graduation cap and gown. He was trying to catch up on his classes. Then a meeting was called with Lance, his mother, and six of the school administrators, during which Lance was told that he would not be allowed to graduate with his class. An unprecedented opportunity for international travel was no excuse; the administrators called Lance a quitter.

Lance managed to keep calm enough to declare the meeting over. Somehow, Linda got him to go back to class for the rest of the day. His job was training and racing, she reminded him. It was her job to handle the details. It took calling every private school in the Dallas-area Yellow Pages, but by the time he came home that night, she had found a school that would let him graduate.

Bending Oaks Academy was glad to welcome Lance for the last weeks of the school year and would recognize the credits he had already earned. This was a small school used to dealing with the needs of kids outside the mainstream. Plano "had one of the worst heroin problems in the country," Armstrong wrote later in his memoir, "as well as an unusually large number of teen suicides."[5] Compared to those challenges, Bending Oaks didn't have any problems with accommodating the needs of a young Olympic contender. The teachers were fully prepared to work with Lance and get him his diploma. Even Terry Armstrong came through with the cost of the tuition fees. Lance graduated with his new class at Bending Oaks and went to the prom with his friends from Plano East.

The limousine he rented for prom night came by the Armstrong house early. Lance got an idea. His mother had missed her own high school prom. He told his mom to put on her "prom dress"—a pretty sundress she liked to wear. With his mother riding in the limo with him, Lance told the driver where to go to pick up his date. Together the three of them went on a tour of the city, laughing and talking in the luxurious limo. He dropped off his happy mother at home and went to the dance feeling good. For once, he had figured out something special to give her, to thank her for all she gave him.

SPINNING HIS WHEELS

After graduation, Lance spent the summer hanging out with his friends. He competed in bike events while they worked at summer jobs. His mother was doing well at work, and he got along well with her third husband. Things were pretty good at home, but he didn't just sit around. As his friends started heading off to college, he went back to getting up early in the morning for training rides.

All through high school, Lance had been riding at Tuesday night Crits and Saturday competitions organized by Jim Hoyt's Bike Mart. As a rider for Hoyt's team, he had earned a stipend every month. Much of this money had gone to make payments on his Camaro. Lance kept up the rides and competitions, but after a couple of months it was getting frustrating. Most of his friends were busy at college, and he wasn't getting anywhere yet.

One evening, he and another rider collided while racing at the Crits. They were trading shoves by the finish line. Lance and the other young man were throwing punches before their bikes hit the ground. It took

Jim Hoyt and several other riders to pull the two fighters apart. Hoyt, a Vietnam vet, was furious at their behavior. He believes that sportsmen should never fight like that. He took Lance's bike.

It was the bike that Lance had used in Moscow at the World Championships, a Schwinn Paramount. Lance tried to cool down. He wanted to use that bike for a stage race the next week. He went to Hoyt's house later that day and asked if he could have the bike back. Hoyt told him to come to his office the next day if he wanted to talk.

Lance just couldn't find it in himself to come around and apologize. A few nights later, Lance and his friends were driving home from a nightclub at top speed. The police followed them, of course. Lance and his friends got a little ahead, left the car in a field, and took off. The police came knocking on Jim Hoyt's door at three in the morning. Legally, it was his car, as his name was on all the papers, though Lance had made the payments. A week later, Hoyt was at the police station working on a bicycle safety program when he was arrested for the outstanding speeding tickets on the Camaro. Hoyt got that cleared up and brought the car home. He let Linda Armstrong know that Lance had to talk to him to get his car back.

It was clear to Lance that Hoyt was trying to get his attention, to get him to apologize for bad behavior and dangerous driving. It's worth noting as well that Lance's mother didn't intervene with Hoyt to speak up for her son. In the past, she had gone to court against the truck driver who ran Lance off the road and stomped on his bike. She'd stood up to school administrators who called Lance a quitter. And yet she didn't tell Hoyt to give back the bike and car. She knew Hoyt well. He had given her good deals on the bikes she'd bought from his store. Lance didn't have to be told that his mother wasn't going to fight this battle for him. He knew it was his own responsibility, and he had to face the consequences of his actions.

Lance was furious, but he couldn't make himself visit Hoyt and put things right. It was almost 10 years before he spoke again with Hoyt.

Instead, he left town. He accepted an offer from coach Chris Carmichael to join the national cycling team. He left Dallas and rented his own place in Austin, Texas. Lance Armstrong was on his own now.

NOTES

1. Linda Armstrong Kelly, *No Mountain High Enough: Raising Lance, Raising Me* (Waterville, ME: Thorndike Press, 2005), p. 260.

2. Lance Armstrong, foreword to Kelly, *No Mountain High Enough*, p. 17.

3. Kelly, *No Mountain High Enough*, p. 260.

4. Randall Munroe, "11th Grade," http://xkcd.com/519/.

5. Lance Armstrong with Sally Jenkins, *It's Not About the Bike: My Journey Back to Life* (New York: Berkeley, 2000), p. 21.

Chapter 4

CYCLES AND LIFE CYCLES

Lance Armstrong emerged as a young professional rider in 1989. His aggressive style of racing got him noticed at the Junior World Championships in Moscow. It earned him more attention a few months later riding for the U.S. national team at Girona in Spain. Aggression wasn't enough to win races, though. "Winning is about heart, not just legs," Armstrong came to realize. "It's got to be in the right place."[1]

OUT FRONT

In the first kilometer of the road race in Moscow, Armstrong broke away from the pack. He rode in front of the peloton, with only one young Russian rider in front with him. They alternated in taking the lead, until the last sprint of the race when other riders had the strength to pass and finish ahead of them.

In Girona, he was in the lead for the entire race, which astonished everyone. Amazingly, Armstrong held the lead until the final lap. And then he lost, as competitors who had been riding in his wake attacked and passed him, crossing the finish line ahead of Armstrong.

The race in Girona in 1989 marked a turning point in Armstrong's career. Nothing was the same after this race. His coach, Chris Carmichael, had told him to let other riders go in front and tire themselves out while he drafted behind them. But once again, Armstrong sprang into action instead. He was seen not as a fool, but as a young competitor who could challenge the best experienced cyclists.

It was no secret now in the racing world that Armstrong was a very strong rider in that race full of world-class riders. "Now, everybody knows who you are, so you've got to up your game and realize that there's a whole mental aspect to this," Carmichael told him. "Until you understand how the intricacies of bike racing work, you're never going to be able to win a world championship or an Olympic Games."[2] He would have won the 1989 race in Girona by using a few very basic tactics.

FOCUS AND CONCENTRATION

"Lance's performance in Moscow was one of the first signs that he was the most talented emerging cyclist in the world," observed cyclist Dede Demet, who later married cyclist Michael Barry. She considered this young Texan to be very aggressive and brash, still a kid who loved to race and never hesitated to dominate any group of people. "After his first year in the sport, he earned the nickname 'King': this is what he was called by both those who revered his talent and drive, as well as those who loathed his brash behavior."[3]

When someone competes professionally, the sport can come to dominate his or her entire life. Every waking hour is filled with thoughts of the sport. Even family members are affected the same way, drawn into that focus on the sport. Armstrong's mother made a habit of reading *Velo* magazine, for instance, to keep up with current events in bike racing and the people involved.

To become the best, many athletes are self-focused. Armstrong had seen what concentrating on work did for his mother, bringing her up the ranks from dead-end jobs to success in business. He applied the necessary concentration to his own pursuits. This self-focus wasn't appreciated by everyone, but it did earn him the respect of many people in the cycling world. Coaches, sponsors, and competitors watched him fight his way through the peloton to the front for most of every race, even though other riders conserved their strength till the final moments and then won.

"He blew nearly every race apart with his attacking style and had a burning desire to win at all costs," was Dede Demet-Barry's opinion. She spent time with Armstrong from 1989 to 1993, during national team events. She knew there were two sides to this young man. "He was both an obsessive competitor, but also a laid-back kid from Texas who always enjoyed a Shriner Bock and good tunes."[4]

Chris Carmichael was the coach who decided to take Armstrong onto the American national team. He was a former Olympian who had raced under director Jim Ochowicz. Carmichael had an idea of what he was getting into with this young hooligan of a rider. He didn't choose Armstrong because of how he won races. He chose him because of how he lost them—trying hard and riding full-out. Carmichael believed that with training, Armstrong could learn how to make tactical use of all that raw strength and willful spirit. He wanted to teach Armstrong how to apply strategy instead of just brute force and ignorance.

During an 11-day stage race in Italy in 1991, Armstrong was riding for the American national team. He was also a member of the Subaru professional team, and their coach asked him to hold back and assist another American cyclist to win. It was a sports heritage and a courtesy, but he wouldn't do it. With Coach Carmichael's approval, Armstrong rode to win, angering the Italian fans. Several fans littered the road with tacks and glass, shouting abuse at this upstart—at any American in the lead. But he kept on. By the time Armstrong won this race, the Settimana Bergamasca, the fans were cheering. At this point, he knew how to win a race but he had much to learn about racing as part of a team and among worthy opponents. Many people saw his confidence as arrogance.

FIRST RACE AS A PROFESSIONAL

"I rode miserably as an inexperienced hothead in the 1992 Barcelona Games,"[5] Armstrong said of his first time in the Olympic Games. Finishing 14th in the road race was disappointing for Armstrong. But it got him noticed by Jim Ochowicz, the director of a professional team sponsored by Motorola. "Och" signed Armstrong onto the team. Now he was officially a professional cyclist on a professional team. His roommates on the team were veteran cyclists Steve Bauer, who had already become a legend, and Sean Yates. The contract took Armstrong to Europe for a series of races.

The first was the Clásica de San Sebastián in Spain. On the day of the race it was pouring rain and bitterly cold. The route took the cyclists 227 kilometers (141 miles) through the mountains, with a punishing climb near the end. Fifty riders dropped out as the rain kept pounding. Armstrong finished dead last, almost half an hour behind the winner. The last of the crowd laughed and jeered at him. It was the most sobering race he'd ever had.

Two days later, Armstrong raced in a five-day stage race, the Tour of Galicia in northern Spain. While he didn't win this race, it was a chance to find his place in the peloton of racers. He got stronger each day, learning techniques for a finishing sprint, and won the fourth stage.

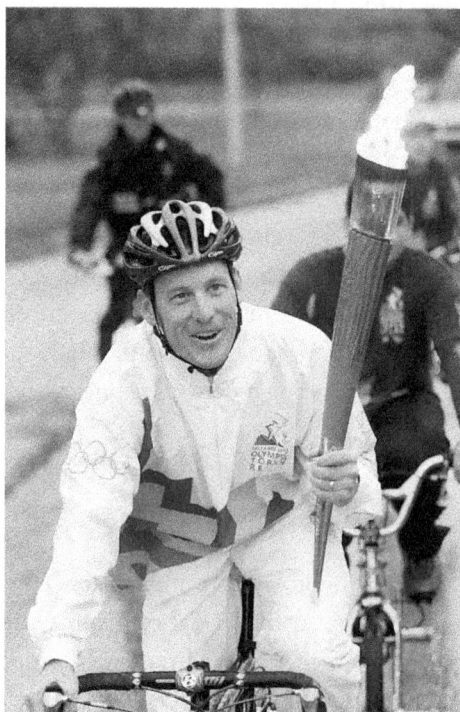

Torchbearer Lance Armstrong carries the Olympic Flame during the 2002 Salt Lake Olympic Torch Relay in Austin, Texas, December 11, 2001. (AP Photo/Todd Warshaw/Pool)

His final standing was 14th, just three seconds behind Johan Bruyneel, a racer for the top Spanish team.

At the airport, he considered flying back to the United States. But Coach Carmichael convinced him on the phone that he'd learn more from the San Sebastián race than any other he'd ever do. He praised Armstrong for finishing and proving to his new teammates that he wasn't a quitter. The Tour of Galicia had taught him a lot, too. So Armstrong took a plane to his next race, in Zürich, Switzerland.

At the Championship of Zürich race, he finished second. Armstrong stood on the medal podium with relief rather than elation. "Okay," he said to himself. "I think I can do this after all."[6]

LAST IS NOT WORST

Finishing last in a field of top-level competitors at Moscow was not the end of Armstrong's career. Losing at Girona did not lose him the respect of his colleagues. Finishing last at San Sebastián brought positive attention to Lance Armstrong early in his professional career. Cyclists and their coaches take note of competitors who are too tough to quit a race. They notice who manages to finish, even at the back of the pack.

"The Lanterne Rouge, named for the red light that used to swing from the back of a railway caboose, is an unofficial but deeply entrenched cycling tradition, a celebration of those who gut it out, refuse to quit. Recipients earn a bit of a cult following," wrote journalist Jack Knox. He interviewed Tony Hoar, a Lanterne Rouge recipient from the 1955 Tour de France. "Each year, dozens of Tour de France riders drop away due to injury, illness, exhaustion or an inability to finish within prescribed time limits. Simple survival is an accomplishment, which is why the Lanterne Rouge is such a big deal, honouring the one rider who has endured more pain, more time in the saddle, than anyone else." Tony Hoar, who went on to design Rick Hansen's racing wheelchair, agrees. "More people know who won the Lanterne Rouge than who came second."[7]

Of course, it's easy to tell who competed the best on the day of the race. "But winning only measures how hard you've worked and how physically talented you are; it doesn't particularly define you beyond those characteristics," Armstrong believes. "Losing, on the other hand, really does say something about who you are. Among the things it measures are: do you blame others, or do you own the loss? Do you analyze your failure, or just complain about bad luck?"[8]

ROLES OF THE TEAM MEMBERS

A cyclist who is part of a professional team doesn't compete in a self-serving way. He or she takes on a role that is meant to bring the team to victory. The teams that Armstrong has joined for the big international races have usually had nine members.

Each of the various roles taken on by members of professional cycling teams is usually referred to by a French name. The name of cycling's governing body, the International Cycling Union, is commonly referred to as the UCI (from the group's name in French, Union Cycliste Internationale). Any English-speaking professional rider soon picks up a few words in French. While growing up in Texas, Armstrong learned a few Spanish words. As he competed in European events he found that he was learning some French and Italian as well, and even a little Dutch. He had to learn to understand his fellow competitors and the members of his team.

The *domestiques* are riders who are "servants" to the team leader. They take turns in the lead, letting the team leader ride in their wake. Drafting behind another cyclist can save up to a third of the effort. On windy days, *domestiques* take turns riding in front of and beside the team leader, saving the leader up to half of the effort to ride.

The *domestiques* who aren't currently "pulling" their team leader along will usually ride on either side of the leader, to keep themselves and their bikes between the team leader and the other riders in the peloton. They will also try to bring bottles of water to the team leader, moving in and out of the peloton. Their role is helping the team leader hoard his or her strength for that last push during the race's final mile. While he started out as a *domestique*, Armstrong was gradually being groomed to become a team leader.

Some of these *domestiques* work as *rouleurs*, and some are sprinters and climbers. The *rouleurs* are cyclists who are comfortable on flatter ground, rolling along at high speed in a big gear. Sprinters take the lead and set a pace intended to wear out their opponents.

The climbers are cyclists who spring into action when the route takes an uphill turn. Climbers don't slow down on steep slopes. They "attack"—they increase their speed and get ahead of the pack of riders. It's a talent that Armstrong has, and few riders can match. If a rider is going all out, the French say that he is going *à bloc*.

The *soigneurs* aren't riders. They are the support team. They include trained mechanics who carefully measure the riders before adjusting their bikes; helpers who hand off water, drinks, and food at the feed zones and at the end of the race; and masseurs whose hands relieve the riders' sore muscles. They take care of the riders. One of the most stable elements of Armstrong's teams has been Willy Balmet. He's a Swiss chef who has cooked for every pro team of which Armstrong has been a member. Willy would come into the kitchen of a hotel and make the hotel staff feel like a part of the team.

The *directeur sportif* is the manager of the team. Armstrong has always relied on his team's *directeur sportif* to give the best advice for the team as a whole as well as for Armstrong himself. With experience, he learned to take this advice to heart and follow it.

The team equipment is stored in a warehouse called the *services de courses*. There they keep clothing, bikes for racing, spare bikes, and spare parts for the cars and trucks used by the team.

Often when racing at this time in his career, Armstrong was frustrated by other riders in the peloton. "Pull or get out of the way!" he'd yell in frustration. He knew that he and his teammates had been told by the coach to keep to a certain speed around the team leader. But at first, during the excitement of a race, he didn't really understand it in his heart. As for his competitors on other teams, well, it just wasn't clear to him that it wasn't their job to move out of his way. Nobody was supposed to ride faster and get worn out just so that Armstrong could ride at a faster pace. He was a *domestique*, and a newcomer as well. Rivals would annoy him on purpose, slowing down or giving him an opportunity to take the lead and wear himself out.

Veteran cyclists, like Steve Bauer, Sean Yates, and Phil Anderson, patiently showed him that a steady pace was best over most of a race. Attacking in the last part of a race got better results than attacking early and having no energy left at the finish. They and his trainer, Max

Testa, held him accountable for his rash decisions and helped him become a real team player.

THE 1993 WORLD CHAMPION

More than two years of training and competition put a little polish on the rough diamond that was Armstrong. For the 1993 world professional road race championship in Oslo, Norway, Ochowicz and Testa believed the young rider was ready. Armstrong thought so, too, but he still asked his mother to attend this race. She took a few days' holiday from work and quietly looked after him and his gear just as she used to when he was a teenage triathlete.

His team was ready to assist him in this race, lasting 14 laps for 160 miles (about 257 kilometers) total. But this time he managed to stay in the peloton until the second-to-last lap, as he'd been told. The rainy weather wasn't good for Armstrong, but it was worse for other riders. There were many crashes. He slipped twice and got back up on his bike. He attacked at the right time and sprang far into the lead for the final two laps. As he won, he bowed to the crowd, blew kisses, and pointed into the sky. When introduced to the king of Norway, Armstrong brought his mother for the brief audience.

He was awarded a gold medal and a white racing jersey with a rainbow hoop around the chest with bands of blue, red, black, yellow, and green. This jersey is worn by the world champion in every race for the following year. Afterward, Linda Armstrong Kelly framed the jersey and medal for display in her home.

COMPETITION DURING THE
TOUR DE FRANCE

The most demanding of all road races in cycling is the Tour de France. It's the race that Armstrong knew he would have to win if he really was trying to be the best in the world. Throughout daily races called stages lasting a total of three weeks, several competitions are proceeding all at once during the Tour. Early in the race, a group of riders will show by their speed and performance that they are leading the competition. Most of the stage winners and the overall winner will be among this group, called the General Classification, or the GC. This term has come to be applied to the top competitors in other professional races as well. Since 1991 or '92, Armstrong has been considered to be part of the GC in most of the races he has entered.

"In addition, earning a stage win in the Tour de France is a prestigious event in itself," observed a commentator at the Gunaxin Sports Web site. "At the conclusion of each stage there is a podium presentation (with babes) for the stage winner, and the winner of each jersey."[9] Each time that Armstrong earned a stage win, he stood on a podium for the cheering crowd and the news media, and two fine young ladies would give him a bouquet and a kiss.

A yellow jersey is awarded to the rider who has the shortest time and is in the overall lead. Green is the color of the jersey for the Points Classification, given to the rider who has earned the most points on sprints during the stage and is the most consistent rider. A polka-dot jersey is given with the title "King of the Mountains" for earning points on climbs. The white jersey is worn by the best young rider under the age of 25, with the best overall time for his age group.

MULTIPLE STAGES

Since 1967, the prologue time trial begins the Tour de France. "The prologue is a short effort in which little time is won or lost," wrote cyclist Michael Barry in his memoir. "Lance goes into the prologue with the same focus as for a longer time trial—he wants to gain as much time as possible on any skinny mountain-goat climbers who may give him a hard time in the Pyrenees and the Alps. In the Tour every second counts, as Lance learned in 2003 when his 61-second margin of victory was the smallest of all his Tour victories."[10]

In the first years of the Tour, there were no steep climbs through the mountains on the routes. Armstrong tells a story in his first memoir about when mountain climbs were first added to the Tour in the early 1900s. One cyclist who made it to the end of the Alpe d'Huez screamed at the race organizers that they were all murderers.

Cyclist Michael Barry says that riding on cobblestone roads is like "having the dentist's drill in your mouth."[11] Every vibration can be felt through the rider's whole body. There's no way to get comfortable.

Muscles tense up all over. Only when the ride is over can every tendon and muscle relax. Riding on cobblestones during the classics is damaging to the bodies of the riders. "The next day I feel like I have the flu coming on," says Barry. "My body aches all over, and getting out of bed is a bit of a chore."[12]

A special part of a multistage race is the team time trial. The winning team celebrates their victory together, as a team. Achieving their common goal as a team feels even better than winning an ordinary stage. Throughout a race over many days, team members spend all their strength each day for their leader in order to help him win the overall title with the best time for the race. It's hard for all the team members to feel rewarded when only one of them gets to wear the yellow jersey. "But when they win the team trial, they all get to kiss the podium girls and throw the flowers to the crowd," wrote Barry in his book *Inside the Postal Bus: My Ride with Lance Armstrong and the U.S. Postal Cycling Team*. "It is the one race where each cyclist is rewarded equally for his work."[13]

Armstrong noticed when he was riding for the U.S. national team that riders often had to hang onto empty water bottles. There wasn't a lot of money to buy new bottles and throw them away. Coach Carmichael was washing out the bottles and refilling them, to save money where possible. One of the sponsors for the Tour de France is Aquarel mineral water. There are motorcycles with baskets on the back full of water bottles. They follow the race route, zooming around the cyclists. Riders who are in the front of the peloton, in the breakaway, have often outrun their team cars. The motorcycles are handy, so the *domestiques* can grab a couple of bottles for themselves and teammates.

REST DAYS

Races that last two or three weeks will usually have rest days arranged ahead of time. During a rest day, there is no racing. Armstrong is usually riding on those days anyway. Most of the competitors will do at least a little riding with their teams on a rest day. They want to keep active and limber.

"Some riders in the peloton ride for a couple of hours at an extremely leisurely pace on rest days, while others ride three hours or so at a steady speed with some intensity," says Michael Barry about his time on the U.S. Postal team. "I know Lance likes to ride at a hard tempo on rest days. Since the team rides together with team cars following behind, the few guys who don't want to ride quite as hard may hold on to or draft a team car to preserve their strength."[14] Holding onto a moving vehicle is a risky idea, and riding close behind a car isn't much safer. Competitive cyclists face dangers like this even on rest days.

RISKY BUSINESS

Professional cycling is a dangerous sport. During a race, the cyclists often ride in a close pack. One small wobble or collision can cause a rider to fall. Because other riders are close behind, there can be a series of collisions and falls. As well, even when the roads are kept clear of traffic, there are other hazards. Weather can turn a good, smooth road to a slick, dangerous surface. There are team cars following close behind the main group of riders. Motorcycles weave in and out among the riders, carrying race officials, or water, or television cameras. As well, the roads are often lined with crowds of people.

"Every cyclist in the professional peloton has had a bad crash. We all have battle scars on our elbows, hips, shoulders, and knees," observed a teammate of Armstrong on the U.S. Postal Services cycling team. "Crashes are something nobody talks about. They happen, it's part of the sport, and it's unlucky to talk about them. I say a prayer every time I see one, every time there is a near miss, or every time I hear bikes hitting each other or the ground."[15]

"Two things scare me. The first is getting hurt," Armstrong has admitted. "But that's not nearly as scary as the second, which is losing."[16] Every rider knows both these fears and deals with them in his or her own way.

SUPERSTITIONS AND TALISMANS

"In cycling, as in many other sports, superstitions plague or inspire the athletes," observed Michael Barry. "A lucky number can motivate a rider while an unlucky number can immediately take the air out from under his or her wings."[17] Any athlete's performance may vary by 2 or 3 percent even on good days, for no reason that is obvious. Looking for a reason can make athletes superstitious.

The superstitions can be little things that no one else would notice. Some traditional superstitions among cyclists are fairly easy to see. During most stages of the Tour de France, if the cyclist at the front of the peloton stops to relieve himself on a lonely stretch of road, the other riders do not take advantage of his break. He can get back onto his bike and try to get back to the front of the pack. The other riders will not speed up into "attack" mode and try to get far ahead of him. If any rider does go *à bloc* the others will tell him to slow down to ordinary speed, which is still very fast. Sometimes the peloton will even call for a brief halt so that everyone can relieve themselves. New cyclists are told to behave themselves; it's bad manners and bad luck to take advantage at those moments.

Other superstitions take place off the race course. For instance, when eating an evening meal together, cyclists never pass the salt to another person's hand. Instead, the saltshaker is placed on the table where the next person will be able to pick it up. This is a superstition practiced by most of the European cyclists in the professional racing peloton. One of the European cyclists on the U.S. Postal Services Cycling Team with Armstrong in 2003 was more concerned than most people about the salt being passed from hand to hand. He made it clear to the team that salt would not move from hand to hand. Or if salt was spilled, that would be even more upsetting! That team member would throw the spilled salt over both of his shoulders to ward off the bad luck. It's not really a subtle superstition in that case, as that cyclist usually wore a black fleece jersey at the time. Salt could easily end up scattered like dandruff across his shoulders.

Armstrong observes this tradition and waits for a saltshaker to be put on the table rather than taking it from someone's hand. Unlike some riders, Armstrong isn't trapped within his superstitions. But he does have respect for traditions and good manners. He also has an honest appreciation of the little habits that bring confidence to a competitor. And yes, there are some superstitions that he uses and indulges for the sense of connection to others. Sometimes a little ritual or an object gives him the feeling of belonging in the community of cyclists of which he is a part.

For years, Armstrong has trained in France for many weeks before the Tour de France. He's made many friends in that country, including Michel Gamary, who owned a restaurant near Nice. It was Gamary's tradition that at the start of the Tour, he would give Armstrong a small gift. These little gifts became something like good-luck charms for Armstrong, who would carry each one for the entire race. For an athlete little talismans like this can be the focus of good thoughts and expectations. That can be very important for keeping an athlete's attitudes and efforts in top condition, especially during races that last many days.

BIG HEART

The long hours of swimming, running, and riding that Armstrong did as a boy and youth had a lasting effect. His heart is nearly a third larger than an average man's heart. It's not abnormally enlarged or swollen— it's a very healthy and efficient heart.

Because his heart is so efficient, it doesn't have to beat as fast as the heart of an average man. At rest, his pulse is about 32 beats a minute. When he exerts himself, his heart can beat more than 200 times a minute. Either of these numbers is unusual enough to startle a doctor listening to his heart with a stethoscope.

When Armstrong is racing, he and the team coach keep track of his pulse rate. They often agree to have him ride at a speed that keeps his heart beating 160 or 180 beats a minute. That's a rate few athletes can sustain for long.

STILL EMERGING

At this time, Armstrong stood out in any group of professional cyclists, not just for his raw strength but because of his appearance. At 24 years old, he still had the classic build of a swimmer. Sometimes, he felt that he looked more like a football player than like a typical slim-shouldered cyclist.

Eddy Merckx had become Armstrong's friend and advised Armstrong to lose weight if he really did want to win the Tour de France. He would have to lose it from his upper body in particular. Even 5 or 10 pounds would make a big difference. There wasn't much spare weight for Armstrong to lose. His body fat was very low. To lose more than a pound or two, especially from his upper body, he'd have to lose some muscle.

Losing muscle mass sounds like bad advice to give any athlete. But muscles on the shoulders can help a rider only so much. Anything more than what's absolutely necessary is too much weight to carry on the steep climbs of a long-distance race.

It did seem at that time that Armstrong was not cut out to win the longer-stage races. He had a reputation for being a single-day racer. "Show me the start line and I would win on adrenaline and anger," he said. "I could push myself to a threshold of pain no one else was willing to match, and I would bite somebody's head off to win a race."[18]

In his early years of professional cycling, Armstrong won two Tour de France stages, but he had not been able to finish the Tour. In 1993, he won the 8th stage of the multiday race before the *directeur sportif* pulled him out of the Tour as they had planned. In 1995 he took stage 18, accepting the yellow jersey in honor of teammate Fabio Casartelli, who had crashed and died on stage 15. "I know that I rode with a higher purpose that day," he said in his memoir *It's Not About the Bike*. "There is no doubt in my mind that there were two riders on that bike. Fabio was with me." He pointed at the sky as he finished, with Fabio in mind. "I had learned what it means to ride the Tour de France. It's not about the bike. It's a metaphor for life, not only the longest race in the world but also the most exalting and heartbreaking and potentially tragic. . . . It is a test. It tests you physically, it tests you mentally, and it even tests you morally."[19]

During the 1996 Tour de France, Armstrong dropped out of the race on the seventh stage after becoming ill. Later, he looked back on this moment and realized it was one of the first signs of his growing illness, a few months before his diagnosis. Another sign was his performance in the Olympics that summer.

"I'd gone into the Atlanta Games in 1996 as an American favorite," he said in his first memoir, "but I rode disappointingly and finished out of the medals again, 6th in the time trial and 12th in the road race."[20] There was a reason that even though he was in his prime and coming into his full strength, he couldn't finish the Tour or win an Olympic medal. He had cancer.

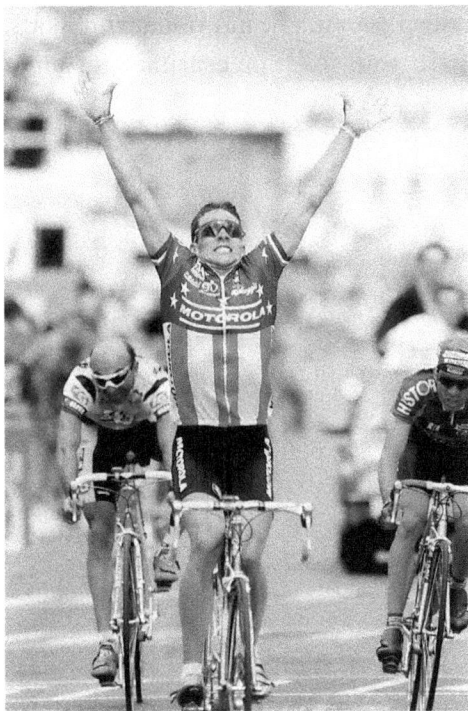

Lance Armstrong raises his arms as he crosses the finish line to win the eighth stage of the 80th Tour de France cycling race between Chalons-sur-Marne and Verdun, eastern France, July 11, 1993. Armstrong, in his first Tour de France, was in a group of six that broke from the main pack with less than 6 miles to go in the 114-mile stage. (AP Photo/ Laurent Rebours)

NOTES

1. Lance Armstrong, "Lance Armstrong Quotes," http://www.brainyquote.com/quotes/authors/l/lance_armstrong.html.

2. John Wilcockson, *Lance: The Making of the World's Greatest Champion* (Philadelphia: Da Capo Press, 2009), p. 91.

3. Dede Demet-Barry, "Lance in Girona: A Look Back," in *Inside the Postal Bus: My Ride with Lance Armstrong and the U.S. Postal Cycling Team*, by Michael Barry (Boulder, CO: VeloPress, 2005), p. 195.

4. Ibid., p. 196.

5. Lance Armstrong with Sally Jenkins, *Every Second Counts* (New York: Broadway Books, Random House, 2003), p. 66.

6. Lance Armstrong with Sally Jenkins, *It's Not About the Bike: My Journey Back to Life* (New York: Berkley, 2001), p. 51.

7. Jack Knox, "Last in the Tour de France, First in Cycling Hearts," *Victoria (BC) Times-Colonist*, July 22, 2010, p. A3.

8. Armstrong, *Every Second Counts*, p. 70.

9. Phil, "Tour de France Primer for Americans," Gunaxin Sports, http://sports.gunaxin.com/2010-tour-de-france-primer-for-amer icans/63721.

10. Barry, *Inside the Postal Bus*, p. 146.

11. Ibid., p. 150.

12. Ibid., p. 82.

13. Ibid., p. 202.

14. Ibid., p. 168.

15. Ibid., p. 93.

16. Armstrong, "Lance Armstrong Quotes."

17. Barry, *Inside the Postal Bus*, p. 100.

18. Armstrong, *It's Not About the Bike*, p. 65.

19. Ibid., pp. 68–69.

20. Armstrong, *Every Second Counts*, p. 66.

Chapter 5

SURVIVING CANCER

Dying young was not in the cards for Armstrong. He spent his youth on the back roads around Austin and pounding along one training route after another, from hills in Spain to cobblestones in France and Italy. When he thought at all about death, he figured that if he did die young, it would be from being hit by a truck while on his bike. He had been hit by trucks while growing up and training. He's been run off the road and hit by various vehicles so many times that he's lost count. There are no illusions here. Riding on roads is dangerous even when there's just one rider cruising at high speed. On most roads, there's always the risk of being hit by a car or truck.

That's what cancer was like for Armstrong. He has the scars to prove that having cancer was like getting hit by a truck. There are marbled scars on his arms and discolored marks on his legs from collisions with vehicles. These scars can be compared to the puckered mark above his heart where a catheter was implanted. Where his testicle was removed, there's a neat scar running from the right side of his groin into his upper thigh. On his scalp are two deep crescents from brain surgery. These marks—all of them—are not flaws. They are signs of survival. They are badges of honor.

THE FIRST SIGNS

The early signs of Armstrong's life-threatening cancer were not obvious. The first sign was simple. For about three years, his right testicle had been larger than the left. Previously, both had been the same size.

The second early sign was subtle. He ached. Not much, especially not compared to the way he usually hurt after a day on the bike. Riding in all kinds of weather on all kinds of roads made pain familiar. He was used to hurting all over. This was just a different ache.

During the winter of 1996, his right testicle became slightly swollen. It didn't hurt any worse than his back, or his hands, feet, and neck after a day's ride. He wasn't alarmed. He assumed that he'd pressed that testicle a little too hard against the bike seat. Or maybe, he thought, it was a natural thing that happened to the male anatomy.

But it wasn't swelling from pressing on a bike seat. It wasn't some normal part of the male anatomy. It was testicular cancer.

After the ache and swelling, there was a decrease in performance. Someone trying to do ordinary activities might not have even noticed such a decrease. But as a world-class athlete in international competitions, Armstrong was used to noticing small changes in his abilities,. He won the 1996 Tour du Pont but was too tired to pump his fists in victory after crossing the finish line. He was completely exhausted. His nipples were sore, which he learned later from doctors was another sign of testicular cancer.

He competed at the 1996 Olympics but finished much lower in the ranking than expected. "It felt like I was dragging a manhole cover," he said in his memoir *Every Second Counts*.[1]

Armstrong wrote that his 6th-place finish in the speed trial and 12th place in the road race were disappointing. It was easy to assume that nerves had gotten the better of him. He also wondered if he just hadn't trained properly for this time and place. His Olympic disappointment made more sense a few weeks later when his cancer was diagnosed. He had competed with a dozen lung tumors. No wonder he couldn't breathe as easily as he'd expected!

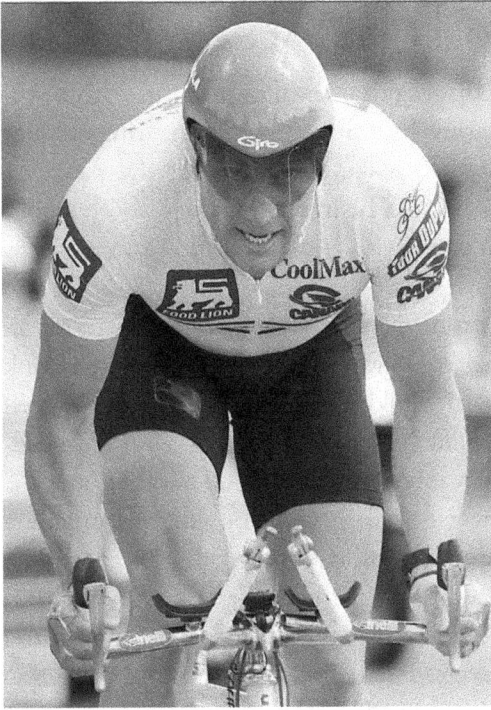

Lance Armstrong races uphill during the final stage of the Tour DuPont cycling race in Kennesaw, Georgia, in this May 12, 1996, photo. (AP Photo/ Steve Helber)

TESTICULAR CANCER FACTS

Some hard bike seats can cause a bruise or a pinched nerve. After treatment, those injuries get better. Testicular cancer is not caused by sitting on a bike seat.

Nothing that Armstrong did by the age of 25 made his cancer happen. A health book on cancer says, "Most testicular cancer may begin as small changes in germ cells before a male was even born."[2] The small changes in the cells may lead to more changes and cancer after a male matures after puberty.

Some researchers think those first small changes could be caused by exposure to something that damages DNA in the testicular cells in a male fetus or infant. The damage might be caused by toxins in moldy grain, or chemicals in plastic that mimic human hormones, or other factors. Good prenatal care for women reduces the future risk of testicular cancer in their sons.

THE WORST HEADACHE

Armstrong had a party with his friends a few days after his 25th birthday. At that time he was dating Lisa Shiels, an engineering student from the University of Texas. To make margaritas for the party, he rented a machine. That day he told his mother he was the happiest man in the world. Later, he went with friends to an outdoor Jimmy Buffett concert.

During the concert, Armstrong developed a headache. It wasn't an ordinary sort of headache that goes away after two aspirin and a drink of water. It got worse, and he tried taking two ibuprofen tablets as well as the aspirin. If drinking tequila margaritas caused this kind of headache, Armstrong thought, he resolved never to drink another one.

The headache got even worse. Bill Stapleton's wife had migraine medication in her purse. Three of those pills didn't do any good. The headache became so intense that he left the concert, went home, and lay in the dark. Eventually he fell asleep, exhausted from pain. In the morning the headache was gone. Puttering around making coffee, he noticed his vision was a little blurry. He rationalized this as maybe a sign of getting older and needing glasses.

This blurred vision, however, was a warning that he should not have ignored. Nor should he have ignored the worst headache in his life. A handful of pills wasn't the answer. These are warning signs of a problem that needs a doctor's attention. Sometimes a headache like this or blurred vision is caused by things that can be treated and solved easily. Sometimes the cause is life-threatening, as it was for Armstrong.

Pain had been a familiar thing since he was a boy, familiar in a way in which it isn't for most people. He wasn't used to the idea of running to the doctor to find out what was causing pain. Most of the time when he hurt, he knew exactly what he had done that caused the pain. Usually he had ridden his bike hard and strained his muscles, or fallen and had an injury. Because he was used to handling these kinds of pain, he thought he was handling the headache, blurred vision, and slightly swollen testicle properly. But he was wrong.

That weekend he went to a bike event in Beaverton, Oregon. Some people from Nike were designing shoes especially for him, and he had committed to ride with them. He was tired and didn't really want to go, but he kept his word. He was finding it harder to keep up with all his plans.

CALLING THE DOCTOR

Armstrong put off calling a doctor for a couple more days. It wasn't like he didn't know a doctor, or there weren't any doctors nearby. His good friend Rick Parker was both his personal physician and a neighbor. A few days later when Armstrong finally called, Dr. Parker came at once. Armstrong had coughed up blood.

He'd also rinsed most of it down the sink before Dr. Parker got there. It was too disgusting and scary to look at or think about. Dr. Parker looked down his throat and up his nose with a flashlight. It might be bleeding from his sinuses, they agreed. Armstrong suffered terribly from allergies and sinus troubles caused by pollen. He never took allergy medication, because it was forbidden for athletes being tested for performance-enhancing drugs.

Allergies could have caused a little bleeding from the sinuses. But the mouthfuls of clotting blood that Armstrong had coughed up were from something more serious. Still, he didn't want to admit that he could have a serious problem.

A couple of days later, Armstrong rode a little scooter through the neighborhood to have dinner with Dr. Parker and his wife. His right testicle was swollen more now, to the point where there was no comfortable position to sit on the scooter or on a dining room chair. Yet Armstrong said nothing about it to the man who was not only his doctor but his friend as well. He didn't want anyone to think of him as a complainer.

The next morning his testicle was swollen almost as big as an orange. That morning's training ride was very uncomfortable. Armstrong rode standing up the whole way. As soon as he got back home, he called the Parkers and told his friend that his testicle was swollen.

Dr. Parker insisted that he see a specialist, local urologist Jim Reeves, that very afternoon. Both doctors suspected that Armstrong might have a torsion of the testicle, a twisting injury that causes painful swelling. If treated quickly, it's not dangerous. If ignored, the testicle could end up needing to be removed.

A quick examination alarmed Dr. Reeves, but he didn't show it. He said only that he was sending Armstrong across the street to have an ultrasound test done. The radiologists did a chest X-ray as well, which scared Armstrong. His friend Rick Parker came to meet him at Dr Reeves's office. There, Dr. Reeves explained that it looked like Armstrong had testicular cancer that had spread to his lungs. They scheduled surgery for 7:00 the next morning to remove the testicle. With information and encouragement from both doctors, Armstrong tried to take in this news. He was going to have many tests and blood work and surgery. He would see a cancer specialist, Dr. Youman, an oncologist based in Austin. There would be no delay in treatment.

He was able to drive home, slowly. He called his agent, Bill Stapleton, sick at heart with worry. At home, he answered a call from a Nike representative, Scott MacEachern, who had become a friend. While talking with Scott the news really sank in for Armstrong. He had cancer. He might never race again. He had to tell his sponsors and his new team. He might even die.

THE DIAGNOSIS

On October 2, 1996, at age 25, Armstrong was diagnosed with stage three testicular cancer. He learned that the cancer had already spread (or metastasized) to his lungs and abdomen. The next morning, he had surgery: an orchiectomy that removed his right testicle. Two days later, he made a deposit at a sperm bank, in case the treatments affected his fertility.

Monday morning saw him at a press conference to announce that he was being treated for testicular cancer. Officials from his new team, Cofidis, made a supportive statement by phone for the press. That afternoon, he had his first chemotherapy treatment. A few days later, he had an MRI scan. It showed two grape-sized lesions in his brain where the cancer had spread.

It was a rough week, Armstrong realized. He got through it with the help of his family and friends. His agent; his team manager, Jim Ochowicz; and his coach, Chris Carmichael, were there as well.

WHAT IT MEANS

At the time he was diagnosed, Armstrong knew almost nothing about cancer. One of the first friends he told didn't know much either, but he did an Internet search on testicular cancer. He downloaded and printed out everything he could find and brought it to Armstrong's house. Armstrong read it all and wanted more.

His testicular cancer was not a small stage 1 tumor confined to a testicle. It had metastasized. The X-rays and MRI images showed that the cancer had spread to nearby lymph nodes in his abdomen. That would have been considered stage 2, but there were a dozen tumors in his lungs as well, looking like white balls on an X-ray of his chest. The doctors called it stage 3.

Blood tests showed elevated levels of HCG (human chorionic gonadotropin) and LDH (lactate dehydrogenase). There were three different forms of cancer in his body, which can happen in advanced cases. The most malignant of the cancers was choriocarcinoma. This form of cancer spreads very aggressively, and cancer cells are carried in the blood. A series of chemotherapy treatments would begin within a week.

"Cancer is smart," said Armstrong, who read stacks of books and articles about cancer treatment just after his diagnosis. "It's aggressive. It has tactics it can change and ways it can resist. When I raced, I said, 'Whatever it takes to win.' Well, this whole thing is just that: Whatever it takes."[3]

At this point, the prognosis was not good. Armstrong's chance of survival was less than 40 percent, said his doctors shortly after the first surgery. Weeks later, the doctors admitted privately that at that point their expectations had actually been much lower.

HEALTH INSURANCE

It wasn't only the doctors who had low expectations for his future. The hospital sent Armstrong a note about a week after his diagnosis, advising him that he had no health insurance. His coverage with team Motorola had just ended when he signed on with the French cycling team Cofidis. The officials from team Cofidis stated that their insurance would not cover preexisting conditions.

Bill Stapleton, as Armstrong's agent and lawyer, argued with Cofidis lawyers that a condition that hadn't been diagnosed wasn't the same as a preexisting condition. They talked a lot but without a resolution.

Armstrong had just signed a two-year contract with Cofidis for $2.5 million. Days later, it looked like he would never be able to race again. He was shattered to learn that Cofidis denied him insurance coverage for his health care. Contrary to what Cofidis representatives had just said for all to hear at the press conference, they would not stand by him during his treatment. They wouldn't help him return to racing.[4]

Trying to prepare for instant retirement with no income, Armstrong sold his Porsche. Some of the art and other things in his new home got sold as well. None of that mattered compared with having no income and no insurance. He and his agent were fiercely certain about a few things for the future. He would get treated. He would get well. And he would race again.

The corporate sponsors who did not abandon Armstrong were Nike, Giro, Oakley, and Milton-Bradley. The CEO of Oakley even arranged for Armstrong to be covered on their health insurance. Oakley's representative brought him a remote-controlled toy car that gave him many opportunities for distraction and play. Armstrong has never forgotten the support of his sponsors. To this day he uses their products and carries their company logos on his equipment.

"Through my illness I learned rejection. I was written off," he said later. "That was the moment I thought, Okay, game on. No prisoners. Everybody's going down."[5] As far as he was concerned, cancer made a big mistake when it picked his body to invade. He was big, tough, and mean. And he intended to win.

CHEMOTHERAPY COCKTAIL

Testicular cancer is an illness for which the treatments are continually being refined and improved. One of the goals is to target the precise kind of testicular cancer that is present. In Armstrong's case, the chemotherapy that was standard in 1996 might not have served him as well as it should. In 2010, the survival rate for most kinds of testicular cancer is about 95 percent, or even better, if the cancer is diagnosed early.

The standard chemotherapeutic regimen for this type of cancer in 1996 was a combination of drugs called BEP. The name is short for the drugs bleomycin, etoposide, and cisplatin (a platinum compound also known by the brand name Platinol). This blend made a "cocktail" that was lethal to many kinds of testicular cancer cells. The drugs are too caustic to drip into a vein in a patient's arm with an IV needle. A catheter was inserted into the middle of Armstrong's chest to put the drugs into his body. He went from the press conference announcing his diagnosis directly to his BEP treatment. There was a week of daily treatments, then two weeks off to recover before a second cycle of treatments would begin.

As many days as he could possibly do it, Armstrong went for a ride or a long walk. As long as he could keep moving, he could tell himself he wasn't sick. The cancer hadn't killed him, and neither would the treatment.

The problem with using bleomycin, the doctors told Armstrong, was that it is also very hard on lung cells. Bleomycin could have caused permanent damage to his lung capacity and possibly his heart as well, which would have meant an end to his professional cycling career. He'd have to make a decision for his next cycle of treatment.

He sought a second opinion, and a third. It may seem foolish to think about preserving a sports career when faced with a life-threatening illness. But for Armstrong and his family and friends, the idea of preserving his health and strength as well as his life wasn't foolish. It took only a few days to find another medical opinion they quickly came to trust.

They went to Indianapolis, where Dr. Lawrence Einhorn had pioneered the use of cisplatinum to treat testicular cancer. There, Dr. Craig Nichols and Dr. Scott Shapiro at the Indiana University Medical Center consulted with Armstrong. An alternative cocktail was available, known as VIP (containing the drugs vinblastine, etoposide, ifosfamide, and cisplatin).

This blend was more caustic than BEP in the short term. Armstrong didn't mind that news. He felt that he was stronger than most people and able to handle pain or nausea. The VIP blend also avoided the lung damage that could result from using the drug bleomycin. This decision may have saved his life. It probably saved his cycling career.

He received his primary treatment at the Indiana University Medical Center.

BRAIN SURGERY

The doctors at Indiana University Medical Center didn't treat Armstrong's brain tumors with radiation. They didn't want to risk affecting his balance and coordination. A slight loss of either of those functions would not be a big problem for someone working in an office job. As a cyclist riding down mountain roads, however, Armstrong couldn't do without his balance and coordination. Instead, Dr. Scott Shapiro performed minimally invasive surgery to remove the two tumors near the surface of the brain. "As good as you are at cycling," he told Armstrong, "I'm a lot better at brain surgery."[6]

His mother and friends saw him prepared and cracking jokes before he was wheeled into the operating room. "We can rebuild him," he said, echoing the boyhood games he'd played at being Steve Austin, the six-million-dollar man. "Better, stronger, faster!"

It was a relief to learn after his brain tumors were removed that both were mostly dead tissue. Perhaps that first round of chemotherapy had had a good effect.

In the intensive care unit after his brain surgery, a nurse brought Armstrong something he didn't recognize at first. It was a flexible tube to breathe into, connected to a rigid tube with a little ball inside. It was a gauge to measure his lung capacity. It looked like a toy compared to the equipment that he'd seen before when his VO_2 max was being measured. He was supposed to blow into the tube, to see if his lungs had been affected by the anesthetic. The nurse told him to blow as hard as he could, and not to worry if he could raise the ball only an inch or so at first.

This simple test was an easy target for the frustration that had been building in Armstrong for days. He snatched it away from the nurse, cussing as he snapped at her that he did this for a living. Holding the tube in his mouth, he blew so hard that the little ball shot to the top of its tube. He told the nurse not to bring that thing in there again, *ever*. His lungs were *fine*.

Treating the nurse so rudely hadn't been his plan, but he saw that his mother was smiling. Linda Armstrong saw her son's behavior as getting right back to normal.

COMPETING DURING CHEMOTHERAPY

During chemotherapy, Armstrong tried to understand everything he could about his treatment. He pestered LaTrice Haney, the chief oncology nurse, with dozens of questions every day. Never a passive patient, he gave her feedback on the effectiveness of antinausea drugs. They developed ways of joking and teasing each other that took away some of his stress.

One month after his cancer diagnosis, Armstrong competed in a classic Texas race, the Tour de Gruene. He wasn't at his best that day. Weak and tired from chemotherapy, he had lost his hair. At least he wasn't alone on the route that day. The man whom Armstrong considers the greatest cyclist of all time, Eddy Merckx, flew in from Belgium to ride at his side. "Hard on the legs, but good for the soul,"[7] Armstrong told a newspaper writer afterward.

A nutritionist advised Armstrong to eat well to promote good health. He was to have organically raised chicken, fresh vegetables, and fruit and to avoid beef and cheeses. Chemotherapy can affect some people by making food taste bad. He tried to eat the broccoli his mother steamed for him, and sliced fruit. Sometimes it tasted good.

Some of the chemotherapy sessions went more easily than others. While the VIP was being dripped into the catheter in his chest, he rested. As the chemotherapy treatment with VIP went on, he found that it got harder to eat much. After a while, apple fritters were the only thing that tasted good. Jim Ochowicz would bring them from the hospital cafeteria for breakfast. They'd eat a couple fritters together, and Armstrong would doze off. A few hours later Och would come back with a plate of vegetables or a sandwich. After lunch, the two of them would play hearts until Armstrong fell asleep over his cards. At dinner, his girlfriend, Lisa Shiels, or his agent or Och would come back with some dinner and visit with him for a while.

Armstrong's familiarity with pain was a real asset during the hard times. His ability to hang on even though it hurt was exactly the quality he needed during chemotherapy. He was used to doing what he had decided to do, no matter how much pain it caused. Nausea was worse than pain in many ways. His treatment lasted until December 13, 1996.

For Armstrong, the familiar thing about being diagnosed with cancer was that feeling of fighting side by side with his mother against obstacles. When she announced that dying just wasn't going to happen to them, he believed her. After all, she'd faced down traffic judges and truckers in court for him. When his high school wouldn't grant him a diploma, she'd found him a new school in a day. Of course he believed her.

"Her belief was my belief," he wrote in his mother's memoir. "I'm convinced that it was that belief, in combination with the marvelous abilities of my doctors, that helped me to survive the disease."[8] His mother reminded him that long before he got cancer, he was a survivor. There were other supporters believing in and praying for Armstrong, even though he didn't know it. His paternal grandmother, Willene Gunderson, saw to it that there was a prayer circle at her church. His adoptive father and grandfather led a prayer circle at their church as well. And his birth father wished the best for him.

TENSION AFTER TREATMENT

After chemotherapy, Armstrong went home and tried to relax. He had his blood drawn every week by Dr. Youman, and the test results were sent to the doctors in Indianapolis. His health was constantly being monitored.

Gradually, his blood counts showed a slow return to normal. His tension began to ease also. He visited his old swim coach, Chris MacCurdy, whose wife got him out in their garden to plant pansies. In his own yard, Armstrong tried planting some trees. It was a process as slow as his hair growing back in, beginning to cover the scars.

Equally slow was Armstrong's gradual withdrawal from his girlfriend. Lisa Shiels had been supportive and caring. He wasn't sure why he'd let their relationship fade. It always seemed that he drifted away from relationships after a while. He had dated his high school sweetheart, and a model, and other girls in the past. He knew that he wanted to be a good husband and father one day, but it just wasn't happening yet.

Every week, Armstrong waited anxiously to hear the results of his blood tests. Were the numbers better? Was he closer to normal? He tried to distract himself with plans for the charitable foundation he was starting. It was called the Lance Armstrong Foundation. It would raise money to support cancer research and people living with cancer. The foundation's first fund-raiser was a ride for cyclists of many ability levels, called the Ride for the Roses.

Playing a little golf sometimes helped his tension. One day he joined Bill Stapleton and Dru Dunworth, a friend of theirs who had survived cancer, at Onion Creek golf club. Needing some balls, Armstrong went into the pro shop. Behind the counter, the young clerk smirked at the cap Armstrong was wearing. It came down over his ears, and Armstrong knew it looked kind of goofy. But he wasn't supposed to get sunburned, so he wore it.

The clerk asked if he was going to wear that hat. Armstrong answered tersely, yes. The clerk asked if he thought it was warm out there.

That was all the smart-aleck attitude Armstrong could take. He tore off the hat, showing his hairless, scarred head. He leaped over the counter, and the clerk backed away. "You see these ****ing scars?" he demanded. "That's why I'm going to wear that hat. Because I have cancer."[9] The hat went back on. Trembling with anger, he stalked out of the pro shop.

Tension was a problem.

REMISSION

After a few months of tests, Armstrong's blood counts were normal. LaTrice Haney, the oncology nurse who had put up with a million questions and smart-aleck remarks from her know-it-all patient, was glad to be able to give him the news. A year after his diagnosis, his doctors were able to confirm that his cancer was in complete remission.

Remission is a very important thing for cancer survivors. It means that there is no sign of cancer cells at all. This was a day to celebrate!

There was something else to celebrate as well, a new relationship beginning with Kristin Richard. Everyone called her Kik (pronounced *keek*).

Every year for five years, when he was tested and shown to be still in remission, Armstrong celebrated the good news with his family and friends. Kristin called the anniversary of his diagnosis carpe diem day. In Latin, carpe diem means seize the day.

He still celebrates that anniversary years later, but with less fuss and formality. It's like another birthday—a day to recognize that *another* year has passed, and life is going on with new goals and achievements.

MOVING ON

What to do right then wasn't immediately obvious to Armstrong. He took some time to get the new charitable foundation under way. He rode a little, because it was a daily habit. A vacation seemed in order, so he and Kristin visited Europe for a while. They went to Lake Como and other beautiful places, staying in fine hotels.

"What I didn't and couldn't address at the time was the prospect of life," Armstrong realized later. "Once you figure out you're going to live, you have to decide how to, and that's not an uncomplicated matter. You ask yourself: now that I know I'm not going to die, what will I do? What's the highest and best use of myself? These things aren't linear, they're a mysterious calculus. For me the best use of myself has been to race in the Tour de France, the most grueling sporting event in the world."[10]

At that moment, stepping into an unknown future, he did know one thing he wanted. He asked Kristin to marry him, and she said yes. Kik was a very confident young woman who came from a well-off family. She knew that she wanted to marry Armstrong, even if they didn't know how long his remission would last.

By January 1998, Armstrong was training seriously for racing. He and Kristin moved to France so that they could live together while he raced for the U.S. Postal Services Cycling Team.

Looking back on a life filled with training and self-improvement, one day blends into the next. Even a season can be hard to remember as distinct from any other. But there was a pivotal week in Armstrong's

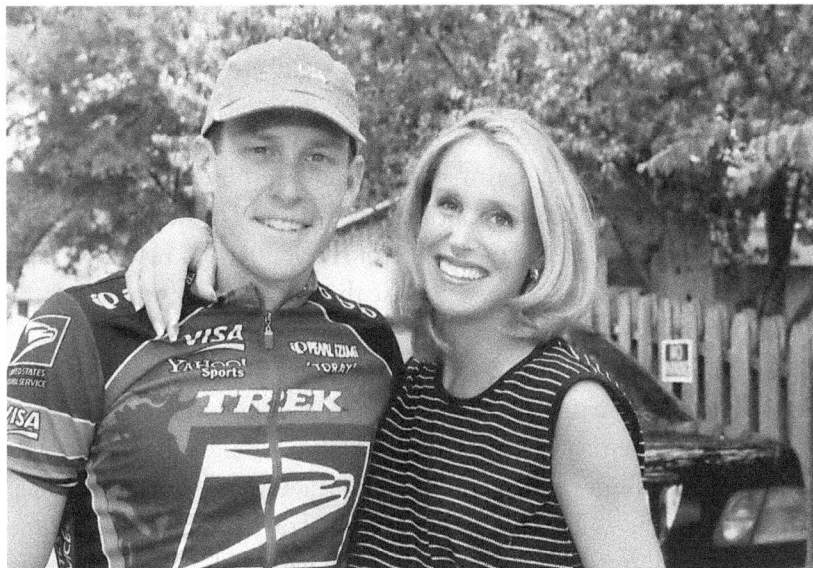

Champion cyclist Lance Armstrong is shown with his wife, Kristin, in Austin, Texas, October 8, 1999. (AP Photo/Harry Cabluck)

comeback from cancer, in April 1998 when he spent a week training in Boone, North Carolina. He rode the challenging Appalachian hills with his friend Bob Roll, feeling his strength return as they raced each other.

NEW BODY SHAPE

Some of the lasting effects of cancer and chemotherapy were visible at a glance to someone who had known Armstrong before his illness. He'd lost weight, both muscle and the small percentage of fat he had previously maintained.

Within months of ending chemotherapy, Armstrong began to look well. Gradually, he increased his activities and came to feel strong. Almost as soon as he was in remission, he began training to recover his strength. In some ways, it was like being a kid again. As he rode more, he grew stronger. The effort and fatigue built new muscles in proportions based on his activities. As he rebuilt his athlete's muscles, he no longer had the shoulder-heavy proportions of a swimmer. His upper body now carried less weight than before—about 20 pounds or nearly

10 kilograms less. He now had the slimmer build expected of a competitive cyclist.

Another change was that now Armstrong seemed to have a deeper understanding of why it seemed to matter so much to him to train hard. Having been exhausted and in pain because of illness, he now faced fatigue and pain and tedious routines once again. This time the choice was voluntary. From the experiences of his youth, he knew how hard training was. He had no illusions that this time around would be any easier. There was an alternative, but he didn't choose to stay retired.

"Suffering, I was beginning to think, was essential to a good life, and as inextricable from such a life as bliss. It's a great enhancer," Armstrong wrote in *Every Second Counts*. "It might last a minute, or a month, but eventually it subsides, and when it does, something else takes its place, and maybe that thing is a greater space. For happiness. Each time I encountered suffering, I believed that I grew, and further defined my capacities—not just my physical ones, but my interior ones as well, for contentment, friendship, or any other human experience."[11]

COMEBACK AWARDS

When Armstrong returned to competitive cycling in 1998, he caught the attention of journalists around the world. He became a figurehead not only for athletes but also for cancer survivors, and he was an inspiration to many. ABC's Wide World of Sports named Armstrong the athlete of the year in 1999. He was named to the Prince of Asturias Award in Sports in 2000. Sportsman of the year in 2002 for *Sports Illustrated*, he was also honored by Associated Press as male athlete of the year for the years 2002 through 2005. The BBC in 2003 gave him their overseas sports personality of the year award. In 2003 through 2006, ESPN gave Armstrong their ESPY award for best male athlete.

He won the Tour de France seven times in a row from 1999 to 2005, becoming the only person to win seven times. The previous record was five wins, a record held by Miguel Indurain and Eddy Merckx, riders whom Armstrong has come to know well and admire, and also by Bernard Hinault and Jacques Anquetil.

At the end of the 2005 Tour de France on July 24, 2005, Armstrong announced his retirement from racing. He was at the top of his game and was recognized as being among the very best riders in the world. It was time to move on in his life.

NOTES

1. Lance Armstrong with Sally Jenkins, *Every Second Counts* (New York: Broadway Books, Random House, 2003), p. 66.

2. Paula Johanson, *Frequently Asked Questions about Testicular Cancer* (New York: Rosen, 2008), p. 8.

3. Michael Bradley, *Lance Armstrong* (Tarrytown, NY: Benchmark Books/Marshall Cavendish, 2004), p. 22.

4. Lance Armstrong with Sally Jenkins, *It's Not About the Bike: My Journey Back to Life* (New York: Berkley Books, 2001), p. 87.

5. Lance Armstrong, "Lance Armstrong Quotes," BrainyQuote. com, http://www.brainyquote.com/quotes/authors/l/lance_armstrong. html.

6. Armstrong, *It's Not About the Bike*, p. 106.

7. Nicole Foy, "Stricken Cyclist Puts No Brakes on Living," *San Antonio Express-News Metro*, November 11, 1996, http://tcrc.acor.org/14.html.

8. Linda Armstrong Kelly, *No Mountain High Enough: Raising Lance, Raising Me* (Waterville, ME: Thorndike Press, 2005), p. 260.

9. Armstrong, *It's Not About the Bike*, p. 154.

10. Armstrong, *Every Second Counts*, p. 58.

11. Ibid., pp. 57–58.

Chapter 6

GREAT WINS AND GREAT LOSSES

When Lance Armstrong returned to competitive cycling, Carmichael and Ochowicz did the best they could for him. They believed that he had yet to reach his full potential as a rider. Many of the same veteran teammates were riding together as part of the U.S. Postal Services Cycling Team. The *directeur sportif* was Johan Bruyneel, a man who was planning years ahead for the team. George Hincapie was the team leader. Armstrong's role was to be one of the *domestiques* protecting and helping the leader. Climbing hills was his particular talent.

With his fiancée, Armstrong went to France for training and the first races of the season. Kristin left everything to come with him. She quit her job, sold her home, and gave away her dog. She didn't speak any French. Soon, she was taking a language class and figuring out how to buy food and pay tolls on French roads. It wasn't some romantic vacation. She kept herself busy while Armstrong was away all day riding and napping afterward. But she kept doing her part.

WALKING AWAY

When he first returned to competitive cycling, part of what wore Armstrong down was the hardscrabble days. He just didn't have any interest in going to a cheap, tiny hotel room at the end of a hard day. Training on mountain roads in the rain didn't make him feel alive and strong. It was cold and wearing. After hours of grim work, he wanted some creature comforts.

Comfortable accommodations are not common in affordable European hotels. Christian VandeVelde posted on Twitter a note about one of his rooms during the 2009 Tour de France. "There is a sign in my room that says 'At harvest time, you could have black insects in your room, they are not cockroaches. Thanks for your understanding.'"[1] It's one thing to understand that some insects are a natural part of farming without chemical poisons. It's another thing to try to sleep with them in your room, then get up to ride hard again through the farmlands.

Armstrong put up with rustic conditions and uncomfortable beds for several weeks before he called it quits. Halfway through the Paris-Nice stage race in the rain, he got off his bike. Riding was too painful, too miserable, and he didn't feel rewarded. He asked Kristin to leave her classes in French and return to Texas with him. They left the simple apartment she'd found for them in France and went right back to the United States.

Assessing His Life

Armstrong took a few weeks off, played some golf, and tried to get his head together. The fine racing bike he used was shipped back to Austin from France. It gathered dust for nearly two months. Meanwhile, he relaxed and ate Tex-Mex food. The biggest decision he made from day to day was where to play the next round of golf.

One reality check came from his fiancée. Kristin told him to let her know if he wanted to stay in Austin and keep playing golf or hanging around the house drinking beer. If that was what he was going to do, she was going to get a job.

Another reality check came from his coach. Carmichael came to tell Armstrong that sure, he could retire. But not before the next Ride for the Roses. The charitable foundation he had started was counting on him for their second-annual big fund-raiser. And he couldn't ride in this condition, out of shape and overweight.

Together, Carmichael and Armstrong picked a place where they could go to train every day. Boone was a little town in North Carolina, high in the Appalachian Mountains. Winning two Tour DuPont races along those quiet hills had given Armstrong many fond memories of training and racing there. Beech Mountain was the crucial climb on that stage race's route. His friend Bob Roll, who had left racing to become a BMX rider, came along to ride with him.

At Appalachian State University in Boone, Carmichael got the athletic training center to test Armstrong on a stationary bike. After months of living a relaxed life, his VO_2 max had dropped from 85, an astonishing rate even for an elite athlete. Now it was 64. Many athletes score no higher than that, but it was a lousy score for Armstrong. The test results didn't surprise Carmichael. He made a bet with the trainers at Appalachian State that after a week of riding, Armstrong's VO_2 max would be 74. And he challenged Armstrong to increase the amount of work he could do, pedaling to over 500 watts, a strong workout for any athlete.

The weather was rainy that April. Together, Armstrong and Roll rode along winding back roads. Some of the road surfaces were unpaved and off the map, gravel and hardpan dirt. They rode under hanging tree branches at times, on beds of pine needles. The rain and cold made Armstrong feel clean. Carmichael cooked them dinners of baked potatoes and pasta. They sat around a table in the evenings, talking and telling stories. Each night when he called home, Kristin could hear how he sounded like himself again, joking and energetic.

One foggy day they picked a route that took them in a loop for a hundred miles before finishing at the climb up Beech Mountain. Drenched from six hours on the bike in the rain, Armstrong left his friends behind on the uphill slope. He rode over washed-out lettering, where fans had painted his name across the road. *Viva Lance.* The last time he had ridden here was for the Tour DuPont, and his name could still be read faintly here. *Go Armstrong.*

Following the riders in a car, Carmichael could see by the way Armstrong's body moved on the bike that something had changed for him. Armstrong could see his own life as a whole as he rode up that mountain. "I saw the pattern and the privilege of it, and the purpose of it, too," he wrote in his memoir. "I was meant for a long, hard climb."[2] The rest of the week went well, and his fitness improved even more than Carmichael had expected.

In Gear

Things came together for Armstrong. He married Kristin in 1998. When he took his bike on their honeymoon, Kik didn't mind. They bought a home in France, where they could live during the racing season. He rode the rest of the season for his team and took great pleasure in his returning strength. And at the end of the year he and his wife were able to conceive their first child with the help of in vitro fertilization. Since cancer treatments had made him sterile, the deposit he had made at a sperm bank was used. For Kristin, learning to give herself daily shots of hormones was a great struggle, but it was the only way they could succeed.

Armstrong's cycling comeback began to be a recognized success in 1998 when he finished fourth in the Vuelta a España. "Pain is temporary," Armstrong told a journalist. "It may last a minute, or an hour, or a day, or a year, but eventually it will subside and something else will take its place. If I quit, however, it lasts forever."[3]

Journalists for sports media and news services wrote about how this amazing comeback from cancer had made Armstrong a celebrity around the world. His example became an inspiration for other people with cancer. "Since returning to competitive cycling, Lance Armstrong became the world's most dominant force on two wheels," said an online media service for young readers. When Armstrong set the record for seven wins of the Tour de France, he was "cementing himself as one of America's greatest athletes of all time."[4]

It was fortunate for Armstrong that he was able to meet Johan Bruyneel, the man who at the end of 1998 became the *directeur sportif* for the team, with the U.S. Postal Services as its new major sponsor. Bruyneel was the first man to convince Armstrong that he really could win the Tour, and not someday, but soon. Armstrong returned to riding as a *domestique* and a climber, but after a year the team was built around Armstrong as lead rider.

SHARING LUXURIES

Girona is a small Spanish city where several other members of the U.S. Postal Service cycling team were living during the late 1990s and early 2000s, including Lance Armstrong. When cyclist Michael Barry was writing about his time on the team, he noticed that Armstrong by this point was earning a higher income than other team members but that he wasn't selfish about his luxuries. When flying to compete in a race, Armstrong would invite other team members competing in the same race to ride in the plane he'd chartered. This was a luxury they were glad to share. The private plane meant that they could arrive without being as tired as they would be after a commercial flight.

"We meet at the Girona airport where we are greeted at the door to the airport by the plane staff, and then we are escorted to the plane," Barry wrote with appreciation. "The plane is parked within meters of the terminal and as soon as we get aboard, we are served drinks and snacks and provided with English magazines and papers, which we are all starving for since arriving in Spain. The jet is similar to flying first-class on a commercial flight, with leather seats and all the amenities. But there are no other people, no lines, no baggage delays, or even baggage carousels to deal with."[5]

The first three times Armstrong had been part of a team competing in the Tour de France had been without success. He had lived rather simply then, as part of a team that stayed in cheap hotels and kept expenses low by eating and living moderately. At the beginning of his return to professional racing, he had tried to return to that low-expense lifestyle. It didn't feel rewarding and it sapped his energy, causing him to quit for several weeks. Part of what renewed Armstrong's enjoyment of the professional racing circuit was the enjoyment of a comfortable life. Owning a family home in Girona was better for him and Kristin as a family, better than if he rented a room there, alone for months. When he traveled, during races the team often stayed in good hotels with comforts that sustained him better than did simple rooms. Many of the comforts he enjoyed he shared with teammates. For most of the years he rode with U.S. Postal, he had a roommate in those hotel rooms.

TIPS FOR RACE WATCHERS

Whenever Armstrong and other cyclists were pounding up steep hills or clocking their best possible speeds, there were fans watching. The routes for each year's Tour de France—and many of the other races in Europe and America—were and still are always lined with fans. "The fans lining the roads get there days in advance," says Primero Picker on Tour Johnny's Tour de France Travel Planner Web site. "Viewing a crowded tour mountain stage is an all-day affair. . . . The earlier your mountain falls in the stage the earlier you have to arrive. . . . The upside to the earlier passes is that they typically are much less crowded than the last climb of the day."[6]

It's a popular vacation idea for tourists to cycle through France or to follow parts of the Tour de France on their own. Professional tour guides can lead fans through this vacation experience, but many people prefer to go on their own. Armstrong has spoken about hearing the voices of the fans whom he is passing. "A boo is a lot louder than a cheer," Armstrong observed. "If you have 10 people cheering and one person booing, all you hear is the booing."[7]

People trying to take photographs or asking for autographs line up along the route at the start of a stage or at a flat finish. Early in the 1999 Tour a child ran out from the crowd in front of Armstrong. He had to steer around the child at top speed. The fans start arriving three or four hours before a sprint stage finish and enjoy watching the race action on a big screen. The barricades along the road will be filled with people two hours before the day's race is done. Anyone who steps away from the curb will lose his or her place.

The barriers are not really an effective separation between the riders and the crowds. Fans dart out into the road to pick up water bottles and wrappers discarded by Tour de France cyclists. Once a fan picked up a plastic bag called a *musette* that had held a water bottle given to a rider. Somehow the bag caught on Armstrong's bike handlebars as he passed. Armstrong is just one of many cyclists whose bikes have crashed because fans have carelessly—or deliberately—gotten in the way.

For fans who prefer viewing the finish of the Tour on the Champs-Élysées, Picker has some useful tips, such as arriving early and bringing a small folding chair. "Bony elbows help," Picker observes. "Be prepared to carry an umbrella (for sun and rain) and once the race ends don't go home—the best part of the event occurs when all of the riders take a parade lap around the Champs-Élysées."[8] That's where Armstrong has been glad to see his own family waiting for him at the finish line.

1999 TOUR DE FRANCE: HIS FIRST WIN

In 1999 Armstrong won the Tour de France, over 2,000 miles (3,200 kilometers) long. Along the way he finished as leader after four stages, including the prologue; an individual time trial in Metz, stage eight; an Alpine stage on stage nine; and also stage 19, which was a second individual time trial.

He had learned to work well with the assistance of his teammates from the U.S. Postal Services cycling team. Worried about sabotage, the team's head mechanic slept with Armstrong's bike in his own hotel room. Leaving the bike out in the team van all night wasn't good for the man's nerves.

Early in the race, the peloton found a cheerful nickname for cyclist Jonathan Vaughters. They called him El Gato (The Cat) after this member of the U.S. Postal Services team was involved in a collision. Vaughters sailed over his handlebars headfirst and managed to land on his feet.

Armstrong finished the race with a lead time of 7 minutes, 37 seconds over the second place rider, Alex Zülle. This victory didn't mean that Armstrong had proven himself against all of the best riders. Jan Ullrich was absent from the Tour because of an injury. Another top rider, Marco Pantani, was trying to clear his name of accusations that he'd been using performance-enhancing drugs.

The major news media in America began paying attention to Armstrong as the three-week race wore on. "At 27, he became only the second American to win one of the most physically demanding athletic events. Apparently he did it without the performance-enhancing drugs that most Europeans favor," commented a writer for the *New York Times*. "But then, he was cranked in ways almost unimaginable; he had just come through the Tour de Chemo."[9] In shock upon winning the Tour, Armstrong was able to say in front of the cameras: "If you get a second chance in life for something, go all the way."[10]

Victory at Home

After touring and racing to celebrate the victory, Armstrong went home to Austin with his wife. It was important to prepare for their very planned baby to be born.

As Kristin delivered on October 12, he was there with her. Together, they waited anxiously for their son's first cry. The doctors and nurses worked to get the baby to breathe. That was a moment of great fear for Armstrong. Nothing came close to mattering like this, not cancer or bike crashes. That first cry meant more than anything to him. Luke Armstrong had come into the world and made him a father. He resolved to be a good father.

2000 TOUR DE FRANCE: HIS SECOND WIN

In 2000, Armstrong faced a number of rivals in the peloton. Ullrich and Pantani, both former Tour winners, were both able to return to compete in the 2000 Tour. This race began a rivalry between Armstrong and Ullrich that was to last six years. The 2000 Tour de France ended with Armstrong in the lead by 6 minutes, 2 seconds over Ullrich. That year, Armstrong took only one stage, which was the second individual time trial on stage 19.

At the Champs-Élysées, Armstrong stood on the podium with the second- and third-place finishers. Kristin came through the cheering crowd and passed him their son to hold. Baby Luke was dressed in a little yellow onesie shirt, to match his father in the *maillot jaune*.

Defining Moments

Of his second Tour de France, Armstrong said that the first big climb up the Hautacam was a defining moment. "I swept up the hill," he said in his memoir *Every Second Counts*. When training his legs for this hard push up Hautacam, he had carefully trained the expressions on his face and body. "I wanted the other riders to see strength in my attitude on the bike, because there was something dispiriting about watching another rider move past effortlessly while you suffered. The only giveaway to how hard I was working was the flaring of my nostrils."[11]

At Ventoux there was a particular duel between Armstrong and Pantani. The winds swirling through this mountain stage were cold and relentless. That's not unexpected in this location. The name *Ventoux* means "all winds" in French. In the high places on this mountain road, there are no trees for shelter or shade. The rocks are as white as the moonscapes in photos from the Apollo missions.

The peak of Ventoux is where Eddy Merckx won the stage and col-lapsed in 1970. He was given oxygen and taken to hospital. He was luckier than the British rider Tommy Simpson in 1967, who died near the summit. Simpson had used alcohol and amphetamines, and heat-stroke took him down. The death of Simpson is one of the reasons that cyclists are now tested for performance-enhancing drugs.

Crashes While Training

While in training for the 2000 Tour, Armstrong survived two remark-able crashes. The first came in May. It was a hot day in the Pyrenees, and Armstrong had taken off his helmet. On a descent, his front wheel hit a rock, the tire exploded, and he hit a rock wall. Two doctors pic-nicking beside the wall put ice on his head, amazed that he was alive. He was lucky to walk away with only a concussion.

The second crash came later that summer in the south of France. While riding on a lonely mountain road with two friends, Armstrong came around a turn and hit a car coming the other way on the wrong side of the road. In the hour that it took Kristin to come pick them up, no other cars passed. The next morning, a painfully stiff neck sent Armstrong to the hospital, where a CT scan showed he'd cracked the seventh vertebra. Mere weeks later, he began the Tour de France—and won it for the second time.

Olympic Medal

After the 2000 Tour, Armstrong went on to compete in his third Olym-pic games, a feat that very few athletes are able to match. At the Sum-mer Olympic Games in Sydney, he achieved another personal goal: he won an Olympic medal. He took the bronze medal in the men's individual road time trial.

2001 TOUR DE FRANCE: HIS THIRD WIN

Armstrong won the Tour for a third time in 2001. The second-place finisher, Jan Ullrich, was his major competition throughout most of the Tour. Many commentators expected that Ullrich would win, but Arm-strong rode harder than ever along parts of that year's route. He won by the largest margin yet, 6 minutes, 44 seconds.

After his second Tour de France win, Armstrong felt that he was truly in his prime. "I no longer viewed my cycling career as a one-time comeback. I viewed it as confirmation, and continuation of what I'd done in surviving cancer," he told writer Sally Jenkins. He went into the 2001 Tour in confidence. "But in repeating the victory, I made a pleasant discovery: no two experiences are alike. Each was like a finger-print, fine and distinct."[12]

Winning at Parenthood

During the 2001 Tour, Armstrong and his wife were expecting again. Kristin once again conceived by in vitro fertilization. This time, to their great delight, they became the parents of twins. Grace and Isa-belle Armstrong were born on November 20.

2002 TOUR DE FRANCE: HIS FOURTH WIN

The competition among Armstrong and the other cyclists in the GC changed in 2002. For that year's Tour de France, Jan Ullrich did not participate due to suspension. Instead, Joseba Beloki was Armstrong's main rival and the second-place finisher. The winning margin for the 2002 Tour was Armstrong's largest ever—seven minutes.

The weather issue for riders at Ventoux in the 2002 Tour was heat. "I recall standing on the blacktop and it was sticking to my shoes," wrote race fan Primero Picker. "With no shade for the last 6k [about 3.7 miles] it was a severe test for the riders."[13]

During that year's Tour, sportswriter Daniel Friebe had much to say, quoting Armstrong and marveling at the lasting changes he had made. "Armstrong also believes that cancer was 'the best thing that ever happened to him.' Physiologically, it transformed him from a broad-shouldered former triathlete incapable of finishing the Tour in the top 35, into the race's most prolific winner of stages at altitude. 'The ill-ness changed the man and changed the athlete,' Armstrong said in 2002."[14]

That was the year a growing number of French fans were cheering for him from along the route, instead of chanting "Dopé!" Television viewers of the Tour—mostly women in France—enjoyed the sight of

Armstrong with his wife, son, and twin baby daughters at the race's finish.

Recognized on the Road

Michael Barry and many of the U.S. Postal Services cycling team trained with Armstrong in Austin a couple of months before the 2002 Tour de France. One of the many vehicles that passed them on the dusty Texas roads was a huge pickup truck. The horn blared.

"As soon as he pulled in front of the team, the driver slammed on his brakes," Barry wrote in *Inside the Postal Bus.* "Reacting to his aggression, Lance yelled and some of the riders threw their bottles at the truck. The truck driver stuck his head out the window, looking back at the group, and shouted, 'Get off the road you bunch of f—ing pussies.' Lance approached the driver's window, and suddenly the driver realized just who he was yelling at. He sheepishly said, 'Sorry, Lance,' rolled up his window, and sped away."[15]

2003 TOUR DE FRANCE: HIS FIFTH WIN

The 2003 Tour de France had the same first- and second-place finishers as the previous year. Armstrong won first place with Ullrich coming a close second. At the end of the final day, there was a gap of only 1 minute, 1 second between the two riders at the finish line. The team time trial was won by U.S. Postal Services on stage 4.

During stage 15, on the final climb on the ascent to Luz Ardidten, Armstrong's right handlebar got caught on a bag held by a spectator and Armstrong was knocked off his bike. Ullrich did not take advantage of the fall but waited for Armstrong. The race judges honored his sense of fair play, but it may have cost Ullrich the stage, as Armstrong was able to win stage 15.

Trouble at Home

In 2003, trouble was developing in the Armstrong marriage. Separations for weeks during training became a legal separation. In June, the couple reconciled and tried to live together again. But by September, they filed for divorce. Over the next few years, both parents worked hard to share parenting and to be considerate of each other for the sake of their children.

Designer Suits

The jerseys and shorts professional cyclists wear fit close to the body. The idea is that clothing shouldn't catch wind and slow down the riders. In 2003, the Nike corporation designers developed a skinsuit for Armstrong and his teammates on the U.S. Postal Services cycling team. It was more aerodynamic than shorts and jerseys.

"It hugs the skin tight, has a rough feel to the fabric much like the dimpled surface of a golf ball, and has few seams, zippers, or elastics that would increase drag," cyclist Michael Barry said of the suit design. "At the Athens Olympics the same technology was used throughout the Games by many of the time trialists and also by athletes in track and field events. At our early-season training camps, Nike designers measured the riders for the skinsuit, and then took photos of them in the suits on their time-trial bikes to document how the fabric fitted to the body."[16]

Suits much like these have become standard gear for Olympic swimmers and speed skaters. But Armstrong usually doesn't ride in them, and neither do most other professional cyclists. For one thing, the suits are far more expensive than jerseys and padded bike shorts—and those are far more expensive than ordinary T-shirts and shorts to begin with. The suits are also too delicate to survive a tumble from a bike. A cyclist or a cycling team usually finds that instead of expensive skinsuits, they'd rather invest that money in good bikes.

The Gift of Laughter

Actor Ben Stiller wrote and produced the 2004 movie *Dodgeball: A True Underdog Story*. In this popular comedy, Armstrong has a brief cameo playing himself at a sports event. The moment succeeds in combining Stiller's self-conscious style of humor with a sense of the ridiculous. It even brings in a running gag about a fictional extra channel for ESPN, a sports network with more than one journalist who has become good friends with Armstrong over the years. The cameo takes place in a sports bar at the fictional tournament for the national championship of dodgeball.

Lance Armstrong:	Could I get a bottle of water? Hey, aren't you Peter La Fleur?
Peter La Fleur:	Lance Armstrong!
Lance Armstrong:	Yeah, that's me. But I'm a big fan of yours.
Peter La Fleur:	Really?
Lance Armstrong:	Yeah, I've been watching the dodgeball tournament on the Ocho. ESPN 8. I just can't get enough of it. But, good luck in the tournament. I'm really pulling for you against those jerks from Globo Gym. I think you better hurry up or you're gonna be late.
Peter La Fleur:	Uh, actually I decided to quit . . . Lance.
Lance Armstrong:	Quit? You know, once I was thinking about quitting when I was diagnosed with brain, lung and testicular cancer, all at the same time. But with the love and support of my friends and family, I got back on the bike and I won the Tour de France five times in a row. But I'm sure you have a good reason to quit. So what are you dying from that's keeping you from the finals?
Peter La Fleur:	Right now it feels a little bit like . . . shame.
Lance Armstrong:	Well, I guess if a person never quit when the going got tough, they wouldn't have anything to regret for the rest of their life. But good luck to you, Peter. I'm sure this decision won't haunt you forever.[17]

It seems that everyone expects inspirational moments from Armstrong, even in a comedy. For the 2006 film *You, Me and Dupree*, he did a brief scene after the credits. There are few people who are both athletes and motivational speakers who could be called on for comedic moments. His delivery comes across with all the familiarity of a hundred sound-bite interviews for sports television—and with a hint of the fun he was having on the movie set.

2004 TOUR DE FRANCE: HIS SIXTH WIN

No one had ever won a sixth Tour de France before Armstrong did it in 2004. He finished with a margin of 6 minutes, 19 seconds ahead of Andreas Klöden, the German rider who took second place. There was a further 2 minutes, 31 seconds before Ullrich finished in fourth place.

This year, the U.S. Postal Services team won the team time trial. In 2004, Armstrong took three consecutive mountain stages: 15, 16, and 17. No one had been able to take three mountain stages in a row since Gino Bartali in 1948. For the individual time trial on stage 16, Armstrong set out two minutes after Italian cyclist Ivan Basso. He made up that time and passed Basso in style, attacking up the Alpe d'Huez to win. For stages 13 and 15, Armstrong sprinted past Basso at the finish. At the finish line of stage 17, Armstrong came from a significant gap behind Andreas Klöden to win.

Winning the final individual time trial at stage 19 made this Armstrong's year to set his personal record of five stage wins in a single Tour. During this stage, on the legendary Alpe d'Huez climb, an estimated half million people lined the 22 switchbacks. The police took a death threat against Armstrong very seriously. "Undercover officers were placed in vehicles ahead of and behind Lance during his ride, and he emerged unscathed,"[18] reported sportswriter John Wilcockson.

The Gift of Anger

In 2004, cyclist George Hincapie was training with the U.S. Postal Services Cycling Team. On his fourth day riding with Armstrong, they set out to ride one of the hardest stages of that year's Tour route. That stage finished with a steep uphill climb to la Mongie. Their plan was that a couple of times that day they would do the climb. That way they would know it in their heads and in their bodies when it was time to race it for the Tour.

"As we crested it the first time, Lance and I discussed all the negative press and the off-putting things people were saying about him and the team. With each pedal stroke, we both got really upset," observed Hincapie, writing about the terrible effect the accusations were having on them both mentally. The pair had done half the climb when they turned a corner. There on their left was a big shack, old and rundown. "On this shack was written, in English, 'Anger is a Gift!' It was incredible; it felt like an omen. Lance and I just stared at it in utter disbelief. We had goose bumps all over." Both riders were shaken to their cores. "It was almost fate. Just as we thought we were losing our focus, we saw the shack and the saying, and we both looked at each other and said, 'We need to get it together!' We both felt the endorphins, the energy, the anger, flow through us, and our legs came alive."[19]

They were renewed in their efforts to train well. For days to come, they rode harder and harder. They were a team inspired to win their record sixth Tour in a row.

Sixth Consecutive Win of the Tour

As Armstrong continued to compete, he continued to enjoy his pleasant discovery. Each win of the Tour de France really did have its own nature. It wasn't a mechanical repetition of the previous year's success.

"Armstrong's sixth consecutive win should go down as one of the most straightforward of his victories. It should have been his most difficult, for a number of reasons: the quality of the competition, Armstrong's age, 32 and last year's winning margin, which was the narrowest in the Tour since 1989,"[20] commented journalist Daniel Friebe in the British newspaper *The Telegraph* in July 2004. During the three weeks of the race the chief rivals, from Jan Ullrich to Iban Mayo, from Roberto Heras to Tyler Hamilton, made an inconsistent performance.

"In 1999 I was scared of losing the Tour every day; that feeling has disappeared as I've gained experience,"[21] Armstrong said to Friebe after his victory at Le Grand-Bornand. In 2004, Armstrong appeared unbeatable, stronger than ever. He won five individual stages and beat his own records climbing three mountains scaled in either 2001 or 2002. Those were the Tours that Armstrong considers his peak athletic performances.

Time inevitably catches up with all athletes. At age 32, it was natural for commentators to look for Armstrong to show signs of aging. After all, the other riders holding five Tour de France wins were unable to achieve a sixth win at this point in their lives—Anquetil at age 32, Merckx at 30, Hinault at 31, and Indurain at 32. Winning the Tour for a sixth time set a new record, one he commemorates with the name of Six Lounge, a business that he co-owns with some friends in Austin.

2005 TOUR DE FRANCE: HIS SEVENTH WIN

Armstrong went into the Tour de France in 2005 with the plan that it would be his final race before retirement. He made no secret of this plan, telling a journalist, "It can't be any simpler: the farewell is going to be on the Champs-Élysées."[22]

"As Gary Player once pointed out, though, practice not only makes perfect it makes lucky," wrote journalist Daniel Friebe as the 2005 Tour began. "If Armstrong has been truly fortuitous over the past six years it has been in other ways. Would-be nemesis, Ullrich, for example, may be as talented but is also as flaky as Armstrong is infallible in his preparation."[23]

This year, Armstrong's team had a new major sponsor—the Discovery Channel. The 2005 Tour was a triumph for Armstrong. During the first individual time trial, he passed Ullrich but finished two seconds behind David Zabriskie. The final individual time trial was won by Armstrong. The Discovery Channel team won the team time trial. At the end of the 2005 Tour de France, Armstrong was 4 minutes, 40 seconds ahead of Basso in second place. He had achieved his seventh consecutive win.

On July 24, as he celebrated the win, he also announced his retirement from professional cycling. At the winner's podium on the Champs-Élysées, there were even more photos taken than in previous years. Gracious in victory, Armstrong praised Jan Ullrich in third place as a special rider. He called second-place finisher Ivan Basso the future of the sport. Armstrong hugged his girlfriend, singer-songwriter Sheryl Crow, and his mother. His ex-wife, Kristin, stayed on the sidelines, and Luke, Grace, and Isabelle came to stand on the podium next to their father. He gave his winner's bouquet and a stuffed lion to Bella and Grace to hold. Luke waited for the winner's trophy to be passed, then he raised it over his little head. It was a moment of fulfillment for

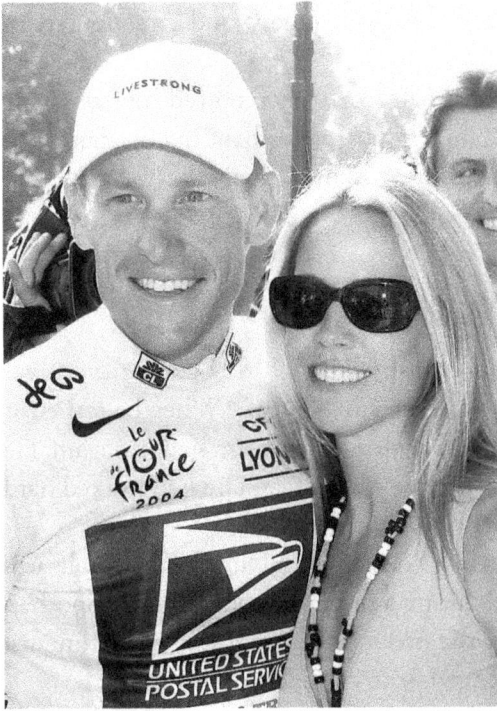

Lance Armstrong poses with his girlfriend, singer Sheryl Crow, as he celebrates his sixth straight Tour de France cycling race victory, after the final stage between Montereau and Paris, July 25, 2004. (AP Photo/ Franck Prevel)

Armstrong, and he felt his career had been completed. It was time to spend more time with his growing children.

A Close Relationship

The moment that Armstrong proposed to Sheryl Crow was romantic. They were on vacation in Sun Valley, Idaho, at the end of August 2005. In fact, they were drifting in the middle of a lake on a small boat. Out of gas but not out of ideas, Armstrong saw this as a perfect moment to ask her to marry him. He'd already bought the engagement ring.

The couple spent months together, thinking about the future. Sheryl Crow and Lance Armstrong came to realize that they cared for each other but were at different points in their lives. They released a joint statement in February 2006, announcing the end of their engagement. A week after releasing that statement, Sheryl Crow was diagnosed with breast cancer. Two weeks later, she had surgery, and radiation treatment was prescribed.

The news hit Armstrong hard. *USA Today* reported him as saying that he wanted only the best for her. He spoke about her diagnosis and surgery on his talk show, "Armstrong Radio," saying he was torn that their relationship didn't work out.

Leaving the Team

"Cycling is a team sport," said Armstrong in 2004. "I could never, ever win the Tour de France without the team. Never."[24] When he retired at the end of the 2005 Tour, he acknowledged his team's efforts again. He had needed each team member to do his best, and he had worked hard to be worthy of their support.

He saluted his rivals, too, most notably Jan Ullrich. Trash talk was something he sometimes did during a race, one competitor to another, but not afterward and not to the press. These were worthy opponents, not enemies, as they strove together to complete each race.

"Every time I win another Tour, I prove that I'm alive—and therefore that others can survive, too," Armstrong said in *Every Second Counts*. "But the fact is that I wouldn't have won even a single Tour de France without the lesson of illness. What it teaches is this: pain is temporary. Quitting lasts forever."[25]

NOTES

1. Christian VandeVelde, "Sweet Tweet," *Bicycling*, October 2009, p. 27.

2. Lance Armstrong with Sally Jenkins, *It's Not About the Bike: My Journey Back to Life* (New York: Berkley Books, 2001), p. 197.

3. Lance Armstrong, "Lance Armstrong Quotes," BrainyQuote.com, http://www.brainyquote.com/quotes/authors/l/lance_armstrong.html.

4. "Lance Armstrong Biography," Kidzworld.com, Kidzworld Media, 2010, http://www.kidzworld.com/article/3667-lance-armstrong-biography.

5. Michael Barry, *Inside the Postal Bus: My Ride with Lance Armstrong and the U.S. Postal Cycling Team* (Boulder, CO: VeloPress, 2005), p. 56.

6. Primero Picker, "Stage Viewing Tips," Tour Johnny's Tour de France Travel Planner, http://letourtravel.blogspot.com/2007/03/stage-viewing-tips.html.

7. Armstrong, "Lance Armstrong Quotes."

8. Picker, "Stage Viewing Tips."

9. Robert Lipsyte, "Backtalk: Armstrong Went the Distance Before This Race Began," *New York Times*, August 1, 1999, http://www.nytimes.com/library/sports/backtalk/080199back-lipsyte-column.html.

10. Michael Bradley, *Lance Armstrong* (Benchmark Books/Marshall Cavendish, 2004), p. 26.

11. Lance Armstrong with Sally Jenkins, *Every Second Counts* (New York: Broadway Books, Random House, 2003), p. 43.

12. Ibid., p. 57.

13. Primero Picker, "Stage 20 Mont Ventoux," *Tour Johnny's Tour de France Travel Planner*, http://letourtravel.blogspot.com/2009/03/stage-20-mont-ventoux.html.

14. Daniel Friebe, "Pain Is Temporary . . . Quitting Lasts Forever," *Telegraph* (London), July 25, 2004, http://www.telegraph.co.uk/sport/2383525/Pain-is-temporary . . .-quitting-lasts-forever.html.

15. Barry, *Inside the Postal Bus*, p. 20.

16. Ibid., p. 144.

17. "Memorable Quotes: *Dodgeball: A True Underdog Story* (2004)," IMDB.com, http://www.imdb.com/title/tt0364725/quotes.

18. John Wilcockson, *Lance: The Making of the World's Greatest Champion* (Philadelphia: Da Capo Press, 2009), p. 339.

19. George Hincapie, "Leading Up to July," sidebar in Barry, *Inside the Postal Bus*, p. 129.

20. Friebe, "Pain Is Temporary."

21. Ibid.

22. Armstrong, "Lance Armstrong Quotes."

23. Friebe, "Pain Is Temporary."

24. Bradley, *Lance Armstrong*, p. 21.

25. Armstrong, *Every Second Counts*, pp. 3–4.

Chapter 7

ACCUSATIONS AND TESTING

There are cynics who say that all world-class athletes cheat. Athletes *must* be using performance-enhancing drugs, insist some journalists and fans. It is hard for some people to believe that the cheaters are being caught. Since the beginning of Lance Armstrong's professional career, there have always been a few wild accusations about him.

"Doping controversy has surrounded seven-time Tour champion Lance Armstrong for some time," wrote a journalist for the *Solar Navigator*, "although there has never been evidence sufficient for him to be sanctioned by any sports authority."[1] Some rivals and journalists insist without proof that Armstrong must be using methods banned by the sports authorities.

MEDICAL TESTING

The International Cycling Union (UCI in French) oversees a program for testing all cyclists competing in international races. The medical tests are not only intended to check for signs of performance-enhancing drugs. These tests show whether the riders are healthy enough to race.

Standard tests are run at laboratories registered with the UCI. Samples from cyclists are tested in many ways, from hormone analysis to checking for ferritin, or iron stores in the blood. The goal of these tests is to establish whether each cyclist scores within normal test ranges for an average male (or female, for women's racing). Cyclists have often worn themselves out during daily training and racing, so it is good to monitor their health. Blood tests can also show use of medical techniques that are banned by the UCI, such as the use of blood transfusions or synthetic hormones. Any rider over the limit of a 50 hematocrit or a 17 hemoglobin, or whose reticulocyte count is off, is suspended from racing for two weeks. The rider is then tested again to see if the results are within the normal range.

There are physical examinations as well as blood and urine tests. The technicians check a cyclist's body fat, resting heart rate, blood pressure, and weight. For high-profile riders like Armstrong, these tests often take place in front of dozens of journalists and photographers.

This loss of privacy is something professional athletes have to accept. "Christian Vande Velde told me that it was one of the most embarrassing moments of his career," cyclist Michael Barry said about these public tests in his memoir. "There are plenty of photos of Lance with his shirt off, Oreo tan lines and ribs poking out, floating about in the media." Professional riders allow technicians from the UCI to test their blood four times a year. The intent is that these tests will show trends and changes in an athlete's blood over time. This is useful both to confirm that a cyclist is healthy, and to show if there are any signs of doping. Barry knows riders who "have discovered health problems that would have most likely gone unnoticed if they hadn't gone through the blood tests."[2]

EFFECTS OF CHEMOTHERAPY

It's hard for many people to believe that Lance Armstrong could be so strong after recovering from cancer without using performance-enhancing drugs. A few skeptics even speculate about the effects of his cancer treatments. Could the chemotherapy he was given somehow have had positive effects on his body, making him a superhuman athlete with stronger muscles and faster reflexes?

Both ideas are ridiculed by Armstrong and by the people who were with him before, during, and after his treatment for cancer. He has made statements, over and over in private with friends and family and in public with journalists. Recovering his health after cancer means he has no interest in risking his health with performance-enhancing drugs.

As well, there's no way that the chemotherapy drugs he was given were any kind of performance enhancer. The cancer treatments made him weak and sick. He vomited all day for weeks, racked with pain and nausea. His muscles shrank because he did less hard exercise. His VO_2 max dropped from the high scores of an elite athlete to a level more appropriate for someone with an office job.

EFFECTS OF EPO

One of the drugs that Armstrong was given during chemotherapy was recombinant erythropoietin, commonly called EPO. This drug is used to promote the body's natural erythropoietin, which increases the growth of red blood cells to carry oxygen through the body.

EPO is a life-saving drug when doctors use it to treat someone who needs it. When given to a healthy athlete, however, it is considered a performance-enhancing drug, because the athlete will have more red blood cells than training alone would make. This is one of the drugs that the UCI tests for in the blood of cyclists. One of the ways to test for EPO or other blood boosters is to measure the hematocrit of an athlete's blood to see how many red blood cells there are. A cyclist whose reading is above 50 percent is not allowed to race for two weeks, after which time he or she is tested again.

Armstrong underwent frequent blood tests during the months that he was being treated for cancer. One of these regular tests was to measure the hematocrit of his blood. His doctors decided when it was necessary that Armstrong be given EPO during cancer treatment. The chemotherapy drugs were damaging his blood cells as well as the cancer cells. The use of EPO was the best treatment, according to his oncologist and the experts in testicular cancer at Indiana University. Armstrong has not made any secret of being given EPO at that time.

After the cancer treatments ended, Armstrong didn't take EPO or other kinds of performance-enhancing drugs. At the time, he wasn't really sure that he would return to competition. He took a vacation in 1997 after recovering from cancer treatments. "I felt as though I deserved a permanent vacation," he said later of that break from competition. "I did take one for a while. I played a lot of golf and drank a fair amount of beer. But that lifestyle played itself out for me after about six months and I found my way back to competitive cycling."[3]

The use of EPO as a performance-enhancing drug is banned not just because it causes an unfair advantage in the number of an athlete's red blood cells. It's banned because that same increase in red blood cells means that the athlete's blood is thicker and is more prone to block small blood vessels in the brain or heart, increasing the risk of heart attacks or strokes. As an athlete exercises, he or she becomes dehydrated. With that water loss, in just a couple of hours the blood can become thicker than it was in the morning of that same day. A number of sudden, unexpected deaths during sleep have occurred among professional cyclists. Use of EPO is suspected but not proven in all cases.

NATURAL HEMATOCRIT INCREASE

There are natural ways for people to increase the number of red blood cells in their bodies. When a person does hard exercise for weeks, the body makes more red blood cells than if the person sits all day at a desk. Armstrong did hours of exercise almost every day as a boy and young man. His body seems to have adapted to respond well to exercise as an adult.

People living at high altitudes make more red blood cells than they do at sea level. Their bodies are adapting to the elevation, working to get all the oxygen they can from the thin air. That's part of the reason Armstrong likes to train in Colorado or the mountains of France and Spain. A few athletes who live at high altitude have been proven to have a naturally high hematocrit. They need regular testing to confirm this condition, and special permission to race.

Another training method Armstrong uses is sleeping in an altitude tent. This tent drapes over a bed and simulates a low-oxygen environment. It's like sleeping at a high elevation above sea level. The altitude tent promotes a natural increase in blood hematocrit. "It's a safe, legal method for doing what EPO does illegally,"[4] wrote John Wilcockson, sports writer and editor of *VeloNews*. Many athletes sleep in altitude tents, especially if they can't afford to spend months living and training at a high elevation.

OTHER ENHANCERS

Other performance-enhancing drugs besides EPO are being used by some athletes. Some of these drugs have a similar effect on blood cells. An alternative to these blood boosters is "blood doping." It's not illegal by international law, but the UCI does not allow it for competitive cyclists.

In blood doping, a unit of blood is withdrawn from the athlete. The blood is spun in a centrifuge to separate most of the red blood cells from the rest of the fluid, or serum. The cells are stored and usually the serum is returned to the athlete's bloodstream. The athlete's body makes up for the loss of these blood cells in a couple of weeks. Then, just before competing, the stored blood cells are returned to the athlete's body. The result is more red blood cells than expected, without the need to increase exercise, take drugs, or travel to a high elevation to train for a month or so. It's a shortcut that can thicken an athlete's blood dangerously. Regular testing of an athlete's blood will reveal if there are sudden unexplained increases in hematocrit.

Other performance-enhancing drugs, such as steroids, are taken to encourage muscle cell development. Steroids and artificial human growth hormone affect the muscles much like testosterone and other male hormones do. As a person exercises, the muscle cells get strained and heal denser and stronger than before.

Doctors sometimes prescribe steroids for people whose muscles are wasting away. Testosterone is prescribed for some men who have survived testicular cancer and had their hormones decrease, especially if they have had both testicles removed. There are other reasons to prescribe steroids, for pain relief, as an anti-inflammatory effect, or in skin cream. Armstrong has received steroid shots for back pain, and they are a part of his medical record.

Using steroids can have unwanted side effects. Overuse of steroids can cause a man to have uncontrolled anger, or make his body stop its natural production of testosterone. In women, overuse of steroids can cause growth of facial hair and fertility problems. The voice may grow deeper like a man's. An overdose of steroids can also cause damage to a person's heart and liver, and even death.

A CLEAR GOAL

It can be hard to understand why Armstrong would compete so hard in international cycling. It's especially hard to understand why any rider would tolerate so much testing and suspicion that he could be cheating. Armstrong seems to have taken on this challenge as part of doing his personal best.

"Mortal illness, like most personal catastrophes, comes on suddenly. There's no great sense of foreboding, no premonition, you just wake up one morning and something's wrong in your lungs, or your liver, or your bones," Armstrong told his biographer, Sally Jenkins. "But near-death cleared the decks, and what came after was a bright, sparkling awareness: time is limited, so I better wake up every morning fresh and know that I have just one chance to live this particular day right, and to string my days together into a life of action, and purpose." He added: "If you want to know what keeps me on my bike, riding up an alp for six hours in the rain, that's your answer."[5]

ONGOING TESTS

"After each race we complete, a handful of riders are tested for banned substances," wrote one of Armstrong's teammates on U.S. Postal. "The race winner, the race leader (if it is a stage race), some of the riders who have placed, and random riders in the peloton are selected for a urine test and a blood test. The selected riders must show up to a mobile lab immediately after the race and give their samples in the controlled environment."[6] During a multistage race such as the Tour de France, for example, a particularly successful rider will be tested several times. Each time Armstrong won a stage, his blood and urine was tested even if a test was done just the day before. All through the racing season, all the cyclists are tested frequently. Sometimes the tests are done at the races and sometimes at the riders' homes or hotels.

"At a random drug test in Canada four of us on the [USA] national team were told by the person testing us that 'they would nail us all eventually,'" wrote cyclist Michael Barry in his memoir. "She then realized what she had said, when we opened our mouths in astonishment, and said, 'We'll eventually test you all anyway.' It doesn't give you much confidence in the system when the testers come across as though they are out to get you."[7]

Each professional team in international cycling is rated each year with points for each race the members complete. Since he first signed with a professional team, Armstrong has been on one of the top teams. The UCI has a rule that all riders on the top 50 teams must have their blood tested four times a year. These are not random tests. All these cyclists must give samples for testing even when they are not currently competing. They must provide their home addresses to the UCI. Every three months they must keep this record updated with their temporary accommodations as well.

Now that mobile cellular phones are commonly used, Armstrong and his coach keep their phones on at all times. They can be contacted when away from home or out to dinner. Any test missed is quickly rescheduled. Missing three tests brings a penalty of not being allowed to participate in the Olympics, and possibly a suspension from racing.

During the 1999 Tour de France and after his win, there were accusations in the press that Armstrong must have been using drugs or blood doping. He spoke to the journalists following him after each stage of the Tour. Under French law, he pointed out, the local police did not need a warrant to search his home or even his pockets without notice. "I live in France," he said. "I spent the entire months of May and June in France, racing and training. If I was trying to hide something, I'd have been in another country."[8] That quote never made it into the newspapers.

THE *BODY* VIDEO

In early January 2000, Armstrong and the Nike Corporation put forth a memorable effort to answer accusations. Their goal was to set the record straight and try to put rumors of possible drug use to rest. "The whispers about the possibility of his using performance-enhancing drugs had never completely stopped," observed Bill Gutman in a biography of Armstrong. "Though he knew there would always be skeptics, he still wanted to have his say."[9]

Together, the Nike Corporation and Armstrong created *Body*, a commercial in the style of a documentary. The topic was the "steely resolve" Armstrong showed while racing. There was footage of Lance riding, undergoing blood tests for drugs, and performing cardiovascular tests, as well as participating in a wind tunnel experiment to measure his cycling efficiency. "James Selmon, the director of *Body*, said he really got a sense of what Lance was like while putting together the footage," wrote Gutman. "The essence of the shoot was to recreate Lance's drug-free ethic of hard work."[10]

The voiceover was done by Armstrong, commenting on everything seen onscreen. Gutman quoted Armstrong as saying in part during this voiceover: "This is my body and I can do whatever I want to it. I can push it, study it, tweak it, listen to it. Everybody wants to know what I'm on. What am I on, I'm on my bike, busting my ass six hours a day. What are you on?"[11]

POSITIVE TEST RESULTS?

There has been only one positive test result among all the tests done to confirm whether Armstrong uses performance-enhancing drugs. During the 1999 Tour de France, Armstrong's urine tested positive for a minute amount of a corticosteroid. There wasn't enough of this banned substance to fail the test. There was hardly enough of the steroid to call the test result an actual positive. The amount of this substance in his body was far too small to have any performance-enhancing effect at all.

When the test result was determined, Armstrong and his trainers made the result public by showing it to several reporters. Armstrong also held up a jar of skin cream. His masseur had been using that cream to treat Armstrong's saddle sores. That was the reason there was a tiny amount of a corticosteroid in his body. UCI officials had been informed about the cream before the race took place and had preapproved his use of the cream.

The test result was not a surprise. It was a confirmation that he and the other cyclists were being tested very carefully. Armstrong did not fail this drug test or any other.

The UCI adopted new methods for testing blood and urine partway through 1999 and again before the end of 2005. These new methods were harder to beat than the older tests. It was believed that if a cyclist had previously been able to use EPO without being detected, the new tests would be more accurate.

PUBLIC IMAGE

In the minds of people who read newspapers and watch TV news, Armstrong has three memorable qualities. He is remembered as a great cyclist, a repeat winner of the Tour de France. He's remembered because he won those races after surviving cancer. And he's remembered because there are repeated accusations of his cheating through use of performance enhancers.

"He may never completely outrun suspicions of doping. The Texan's Tour victories can be catalogued according to the controversies that have pursued him," wrote journalist Daniel Friebe. He noted that the 2004 Tour de France would be remembered for Armstrong's taking legal action against the authors of a controversial book, *L.A. Confidentiel: Les Secrets de Lance Armstrong* (in English, *L.A. Confidential: The Secrets of Lance Armstrong*). The authors, Pierre Ballester and David Walsh, presented circumstantial evidence suggesting that Armstrong used performance enhancers. Friebe noted that this book included a statement by three-time Tour winner Greg Lemond that "Lance will do anything to keep his secret."[12] The authors made much of the fact that the team doctor for Armstrong's team, Dr. Michele Ferrari, was accused in Italy of sporting fraud and related charges. The book's claims of guilt by association were summarized for an article in a London newspaper, the *Sunday Times*. That's when Armstrong sued the paper and the authors for libel. The paper and authors eventually settled out of court.

"Increasingly, Armstrong's protests that he has never tested positive no longer seem to suffice. By banning all riders merely named in ongoing legal proceedings from this year's Tour, organisers Amaury Sport Organisation (ASO), acknowledged that the presumption of innocence can no longer apply, so grave has cycling's doping problem become," wrote journalist Daniel Friebe after the 2004 Tour de France. "Dope tests are so inadequate and confidence in the sport's governing body, the International Cycling Union (UCI), so low that to suggest that Armstrong is definitely innocent would be as irresponsible as to say that he is definitely not." In Friebe's opinion, "Armstrong has been failed by sports authorities who have been unable to protect and prove the authenticity of perhaps their greatest champion."[13]

AS HE RETIRED

Armstrong made several statements to journalists after the 2005 Tour de France, when he announced his retirement. "It's nice to win. I'll never win again," Armstrong quipped at one point. "I may have to take up golf—take on Tiger."[14]

Less than a month later, in late August 2005, the French sports newspaper *l'Équipe* claimed that there was evidence in old urine samples from 1999. The article claimed these old samples had been tested by the World Anti-Doping Agency (WADA) using new methods that were just put into use in 2005. The article stated that the samples showed that Armstrong had used EPO in the 1999 Tour de France. The headline of their article translated to "Armstrong Lies."

For his part, Armstrong denied using EPO. "I do not use, and have never used, performance-enhancing drugs," he said in a press release at that time while on holiday in southern France with his children. "The investigators are welcome to review my long history of tests for performance-enhancing drugs, which I have never failed. Last year [2004] alone I was tested twenty-two times by the UCI, WADA and USADA [the US Anti-Doping Agency]."[15]

The UCI did not make any statements until their investigation was complete. "In response to the *l'Équipe* allegations, an independent investigation was begun by the International Cycling Union in October of 2005," reported Daniel Friebe. "The investigation has reported that Armstrong did not engage in doping and that the World Anti-Doping Agency had acted 'completely inconsistent' with testing rules."[16] The ICU stated that there was no proof that the five-year-old samples were from Armstrong. There was no believable history to show these samples hadn't been warmed up and frozen again several times. There was no way to be sure if any testable evidence would remain after the samples were stored for five years. EPO traces aren't stable in urine for five years, even if the samples had been kept at a constant temperature of $-20°C$ ($-4°F$).

CLEANING HOUSE

The UCI has made a determined effort to eliminate from international racing any cyclists who use banned substances. As new testing methods became available in 1999 and 2005, they were adopted. Newer methods were developed in 2008 to test for the latest versions of blood boosters and other kinds of cheating. The tests done on Armstrong's samples were always the best available. He didn't leave racing at times that would have conveniently kept him from being subject to more accurate tests.

The organizers of the major races cooperated with the UCI, particularly the planners for the Tour de France. "In the 2008 Tour, 180 riders entered, and only 8 were caught up in doping scandal. That is less than 4.5%, and the biggest names were caught using MIRCERA, a new form of EPO which had just recently been developed," reported the Gunaxin Web site on sports. "The testing kept up with the cheaters, and even the newest form was detected. The 2009 Tour de France was able to conclude without being marred by a single positive doping result."[17]

Because of this effective testing campaign, "A revitalized, scandal-free Tour focused more on rider rivalry than on drugs," commented Chris Redden in *Pedal* magazine. "The doping ain't over, but positive steps are taking hold."[18]

Cyclist Floyd Landis made accusations in 2010. Landis claimed that in the past Armstrong had given him banned drugs, and Landis saw him get secret transfusions of blood. These claims are being investigated, even though Landis has changed his story many times. Over a couple of years, Landis told a variety of stories to the press, in a book, and under oath. "Despite the accusations from Floyd Landis, Lance Armstrong has never failed a drug test, despite being among the most tested athletes in all of sports," observed a commentator for the Gunaxin Web site. "Cycling has never ignored their doping problem, and they have always been at the forefront of fighting it. I wish the same could be said for other sports that we enjoy."[19]

WOULD IT BE SO BAD?

One of the things some critics say about Armstrong is that maybe he might not think it's wrong to use performance-enhancing drugs. Maybe he would use a drug because he doesn't believe that it's dangerous. After all, he was given EPO during cancer treatment. That drug might not seem as dangerous as other medicines. Maybe he might think that medicines given by a doctor aren't as dangerous as street drugs. Performance enhancers aren't banned in all sports, they're banned only by some sports officials, such as the UCI for cycling.

Or maybe, some critics suggest, he doesn't think it's unfair to use drugs. Cancer wasn't fair. Maybe drugs would just give back what cancer took away. Maybe drugs would just bring him back to his own normal performance. Maybe he always used drugs, even as a teenager, and it would seem normal to use them. That idea doesn't ring true to people who knew him as a teenager. Armstrong's former swim coach admits that some people believe that to be as good as Armstrong, a rider would have to be doing something outside the norm, something that was probably illegal. "But he is so meticulous about everything he does, and he's such a rare human being, physically, that he doesn't have to do that," said Chris MacCurdy. "Not a chance, not a chance."[20] Scott Eder, a sports mentor to the teenaged Lance, keeps an open mind. "I want to believe that he didn't take drugs, and I think at this point he has proved that he didn't."[21]

It was hard for his mother, Linda, to get her teenaged son to follow the advice of doctors to rest after injuries. She wouldn't have accepted the idea of his taking drugs to become stronger. It was hard to get him tired out enough to sleep. As for what's fair or unfair about cancer, Armstrong learned good lessons about fairness from his mother. To the two of them, every setback or obstacle isn't unfair, it's an opportunity to succeed by trying harder in another way.

Another idea that was suggested during 2010 is that maybe Armstrong doesn't think that rules apply to him. Maybe he thinks that laws and rules are for other people. That idea doesn't ring true. The only laws that Armstrong seems to break are speeding laws in his car. In Texas, that's illegal but not unusual among otherwise law-abiding citizens. He had a stack of speeding tickets as a teenager, but no convictions for offenses such as collisions or drunk driving.

POSSIBLE CHARGES BEING CONSIDERED

One concern for some commentators on cycling is the accusation that Floyd Landis made in 2010. Landis claimed that when he and Lance Armstrong were riding on the same team, there was blood doping and use of performance-enhancing drugs such as testosterone patches and EPO. Landis claimed that these incidents took place while the team's primary sponsor was the U.S. Postal Services.

Even though the postal system does not receive payments directly from Congress, it is still considered a public or government entity. The revenues of the U.S. Postal Services are considered public funds. "The theory suggests that because the team received public funds and then allegedly conspired to purchase, distribute, and use illegally acquired prescription drugs and other substances that it would constitute a misuse of those public funds," commented Charles Pelkey for the *Velonews* Web site. "It could be a valid charge to consider, but there is one huge hurdle in that road, namely the section of the U.S. Code that outlines the statute of limitations (18 U.S.C. Section 3282). That establishes that there cannot be prosecutions for most crimes committed more than five years prior to the issuance of an indictment."[22] At the end of 2004, the Postal Service was no longer the sponsor of the team that included Lance Armstrong and Floyd Landis. As of August 2010, no charges had been laid as a result of Landis's accusations.

Pelkey considers it possible that charges might be considered under the Racketeer Influenced and Corrupt Organizations Act that was passed in 1970. This act allows for prosecution of two or more acts of racketeering activity within 10 years if bank fraud is involved. "Racketeering activity is a broad term that includes just about any nefarious deed," observes Pelkey, "such as . . . bribery (including sports bribery), or . . . chemicals and drugs that fall under the Controlled Substances Act."[23] He doesn't speculate about whether it is likely that such charges might be laid in the future.

TEST RESULTS IN PUBLIC

"I'm surely the most drug-tested man on the planet," Armstrong wrote in his 2003 memoir. That still felt true to him years later. "I'm tested anywhere from 30 to 40 times a year, both in and out of competition, and I welcome it, because frankly, it's the only proof I have of my innocence."[24]

In September 2008, Armstrong announced his second comeback to professional racing. He later told *VeloNews* that he would post online the results of his blood tests, just to quiet the still-persistent rumors of drug use.

The UCI has rules insisting that cyclists must be in antidoping testing programs for six months before to an event. The officials gave Armstrong special permission to participate in the Australian Tour Down Under during January 2009 with only a few months of previous testing. For the UCI, engaging the leading antidoping scientist Don Catlin was an acceptable equivalent. Catlin did independent tests on Armstrong throughout his comeback races.

"I have to be happy. I'm 39 years old. I've been doing this for 17 years and I'm still at the front," Armstrong said to reporters during the 2010 Tour de Suisse. "So despite the things that I read in newspapers and on the internet every day of people talking about me. . . . The record speaks for itself."[25]

NOTES

1. "Tour de France," *Solar Navigator*, http://www.solarnavigator.net/sport/tour_de_france.htm.

2. Michael Barry, *Inside the Postal Bus: My Ride with Lance Armstrong and the U.S. Postal Cycling Team* (Boulder, CO: VeloPress, 2005), p. 145.

3. Lance Armstrong, *Comeback 2.0: Up Close and Personal* (New York: Touchstone/Simon & Schuster, 2009), p. i.

4. John Wilcockson, *Lance: The Making of the World's Greatest Champion* (Philadelphia: Da Capo Press, 2009), p. 298.

5. Lance Armstrong with Sally Jenkins, *Every Second Counts* (New York: Broadway Books, Random House, 2003), p. 8.

6. Barry, *Inside the Postal Bus*, pp. 88–89.

7. Ibid.

8. Lance Armstrong with Sally Jenkins, *It's Not About the Bike: My Journey Back to Life* (New York: Berkley Books, 2001), p. 248.

9. Bill Gutman, *Lance Armstrong: A Biography* (New York: Simon Pulse, 2005), p. 112.

10. Ibid., p. 112.

11. Ibid.

12. Daniel Friebe, "Pain Is Temporary . . . Quitting Lasts Forever," *Telegraph* (London), July 25, 2004, http://www.telegraph.co.uk/sport/2383525/Pain-is-temporary . . .-quitting-lasts-forever.html.

13. Ibid.

14. Lance Armstrong, "Lance Armstrong Quotes," BrainyQuote.com, http://www.brainyquote.com/quotes/authors/l/lance_armstrong.html.

15. Wilcockson, *Lance: The Making*, p. 344.

16. "Tour de France," *Solar Navigator*.

17. Phil, "Tour de France Primer for Americans." *Gunaxin Sports*, http://sports.gunaxin.com/2010-tour-de-france-primer-for-americans/63721

18. Chris Redden, "Tread," *Pedal*, Fall 2009, p. 6.

19. Phil, "Tour de France Primer."

20. Wilcockson, *Lance: The Making*, p. 354.

21. Ibid.

22. Charles Pelkey, "The Explainer: What Crimes Could Federal Investigators Charge against Lance Armstrong?" Velonews, http://velonews.competitor.com/2010/07/news/the-explainer-what-crimes-could-federal-investigators-charge-against-lance-armstrong_132057.

23. Ibid.

24. Armstrong, *Every Second Counts*, p. 60.

25. Lynne Butler, "2010 Tour de Suisse, Stage 7 Results, Burghardt Takes His Second Stage," *Seattle Examiner*, June 18, 2010, http://www.examiner.com/endurance-sports-in-seattle/2010-tour-de-suisse-stage-7-results-burghardt-takes-his-second-stage.

Chapter 8

LIVESTRONG

The first time that Lance Armstrong made a public statement about having cancer was at a press conference on October 8, 1996. When he announced that he had just been diagnosed with advanced testicular cancer, Bill Stapleton was there as his agent and friend. Jim Ochowicz made a supportive statement as the director for team Motorola, which Armstrong had just left. Armstrong described his symptoms, diagnosis, and treatment, briefly and in plain words.

"I intend to be an avid spokesperson for testicular cancer once I have beaten the disease," he made sure to say. "Had I been more aware of the symptoms, I believe I would have seen a doctor before my condition had advanced to this stage. I want this to be a positive experience and I want to take this opportunity to help others who might someday suffer from the same circumstance I face today."[1] This press conference was the beginning of Armstrong's public motivational work.

THE DUTY OF THE SURVIVOR

For three months that seemed to take forever, Armstrong was given chemotherapy. During the last week of treatment in December 1996, his doctor, Craig Nichols, came by to talk with him. This time it wasn't one of what had become their usual conversations. Armstrong was always asking about the nature of the drugs the nurses were giving him. He was learning what the blood tests meant with regard to how his body was responding to these medications. This time the doctor had an agenda of his own.

He spoke with Armstrong about the duty of the survivor. So far, the treatments were working. It now seemed likely that Armstrong was not, in fact, about to die in a few weeks. The doctor believed that Armstrong had to take on the responsibility of a cancer survivor. Though it would be months before the blood tests would show whether Armstrong was cured, he was alive now. What would he do with his knowledge of what it was like to have cancer? What would he do with the obligation that came with being cured? How could he use what he knew to help people?

It was a little like the line from poet Mary Oliver that Armstrong's friend Lee Walker used to quote when they were teenagers: "Tell me, what is it you plan to do with your one wild and precious life?"[2]

What to do with the rest of his life wasn't immediately clear to Armstrong. But he knew what to do right then about his responsibility as a cancer survivor. He held a charity benefit ride, right at home in Austin. He and his friends organized this race. It was a good first step.

ON THE TEAM

That first benefit ride was a fund-raiser. Previously, Armstrong and his friends had been organizing a little local race in Austin on Valentine's Day that they called the Ride for the Roses. This year, he wanted to make it a bigger event. There were three separate races: a 10-mile (16-km) fun ride, a 25-mile (40-km) loop, and a 100-mile (160-km) race for the hardcore riders. Four bands were playing for the party afterward. The ride was organized with the help of friends while Armstrong was undergoing chemotherapy treatments.

He decided that he was going to start a charitable foundation: the Lance Armstrong Foundation. This race was its first fund-raising event. The goal was to raise money for cancer research and to support people with cancer and their families. While going through treatment, he saw that his illness affected more than just himself. His mother and his friends were also affected. Friends who had felt helpless about his illness were glad to be able to do something positive by participating in this benefit ride. The board of directors for the foundation included Armstrong's doctors.

His corporate sponsors, Oakley, Nike, Giro, and Milton-Bradley, were affected by his illness, too. When he called up the representatives from his corporate sponsors to tell them he had cancer, they were supportive. Less than three months later, he called them again to tell them that he was starting a charitable foundation. He needed funding to stage the Ride for the Roses. Every one of his sponsors helped. Instead of being faceless major businesses, these corporations were on the team as the Lance Armstrong Foundation began.

The first fund-raising event was a great success. People lined up to sign in for the race and make donations. Armstrong was at a table signing autographs with other celebrity athletes when a checkbook fell open in front of him and he heard a familiar voice say: "How much do

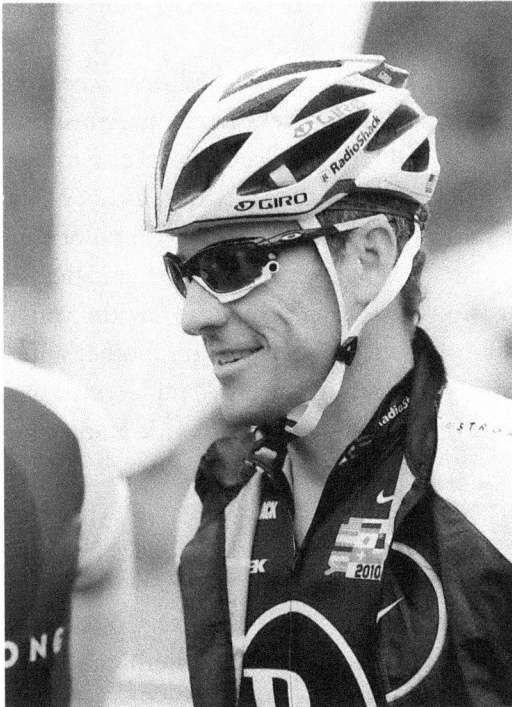

Cyclist Lance Armstrong greets fellow riders prior to the start of his LiveSTRONG Challenge 10K ride for cancer on August 22, 2010, in Blue Bell, Pennsylvania. (AP Photo/Bradley C. Bower)

you want?" "It was the long-lost Jim Hoyt, the man who put me on my first bike and then took my beloved Camaro away," he realized. "He was standing right in front of me, and so was his wife Rhonda."[3] Armstrong said he was sorry, Hoyt accepted his apology, and that was that. Since then, every year they meet at the Ride for the Roses, and Hoyt makes another donation.

NOT ALONE

The diagnosis that he had cancer wasn't an isolated event in Armstrong's life. Just a week earlier, his old friend J. T. Hoyt had been diagnosed with cancer. Hoyt lived for six more years and was oddly proud of having "maxed out" his insurance coverage before he passed on.

As well, during Armstrong's recovery, the assistant to his agent, Bill Stapledon, was also stricken with cancer. Stacy Pounds was very motherly and supportive to Armstrong and had become a good friend. In January 1997 she helped launch the Lance Armstrong Foundation. That same month, Pounds was diagnosed with lung cancer. She and Armstrong gave each other matching cross necklaces to wear as symbols of their cancer kinship.

Pounds quickly deteriorated. Doctors said she had only weeks to live. Care in a nursing home was unable to relieve her pain. Armstrong and Stapledon took her home and hired a hospice nurse to care for her full-time. Pounds's son was on a tour of duty at sea with the U.S. Navy. It took a phone call to four-star general Charles Boyd to get sailor Paul Pounds home to see his mother. Boyd had met Armstrong, and he had lost his own wife to cancer two years earlier. The next day the young sailor was on his way home for the remaining days of his mother's life.

"That's what the term 'cancer community' means,"[4] said Armstrong. He wore her cross all the time he was racing in the Tour de France. He still wears it.

GROWING AND EXPANDING

Starting a charitable foundation was a sensible idea for this time in Armstrong's life. While learning the ins and outs of international cycling over the last few years, Armstrong had been learning what he could about business as well. During the racing season, he was often on the Internet, keeping track of his investments, and watching CNN. He became an investor in the team for which he raced. Starting a foundation taught him a great deal.

The first volunteers and employees of the foundation were Armstrong's friends, some new and some he'd known for years. The first manager of the foundation was John Korioth, a longtime friend and training partner. The second employee hired by the Lance Armstrong Foundation was photographer Elizabeth Kreutz. Armstrong met Kreutz when he moved to Austin in 1990. Over the years Liz has become like a sister to him. Her photographs became the core of a book they created together about his second comeback to racing in 2008.

Working with the Lance Armstrong Foundation introduced him to both of the women who have borne his children—his ex-wife Kristin Richard Armstrong and his girlfriend, Anna Hansen. He met Kristin when she was the representative of a corporate sponsor for the first Ride for the Roses. A few years after his divorce, Anna Hansen was working for a scion group of the foundation and they got to know each other.

There are now so many volunteers with the foundation that Armstrong can't know them all. But many of the employees and board members of the foundation are still or have become his personal friends. The staff includes people who maintain active Web sites and blogs with new content and material from foundation activities across the United States and around the world.

THE PUBLIC FACE OF CANCER

As a spokesman for cancer survivors, Armstrong is more than a pretty face in front of the cameras. He has kept up with his reading about cancer, its causes and its treatments. When he makes a statement about the foundation he began, it's not just because he's a figurehead and a spokesman. He promotes the foundation's programs because he knows that the focus really is on people with cancer. The money raised supports them and their families and goes toward research for a cure.

"Armstrong knows that people with cancer look to him for inspiration from their hospital rooms," says a health book from a series for young adult readers. "He is motivated to succeed because of their attention, and he wants to motivate them to succeed in their own fight to survive cancer."[5]

One of the real benefits that Armstrong brings to the fight against cancer is that he is willing to say out loud that he had testicular cancer. Many men are just not able to talk at all about cancer and their private parts. By making public statements, Armstrong is being a role model.

At a press conference for the foundation in 2004, Armstrong spoke out about how he had ignored his symptoms until it was almost too late. "I am dedicated to the Cycle of Hope campaign because I want to help others break out of their cycle of misunderstanding and fear," he said, "and empower themselves through the Cycle of Hope."[6] His health and strength after surviving cancer are inspiring for many people.

Seeing children stricken with cancer is particularly hard for Armstrong. He's not alone in that. The way that children can hope even when they hurt inspires him. "If children have the ability to ignore all odds and percentages, then maybe we can all learn from them," Armstrong said. "When you think about it, what other choice is there but to hope? We have two options, medically and emotionally: give up, or Fight Like Hell."[7]

MOTIVATIONAL WRISTBANDS

One of the smallest but most successful projects of the Lance Armstrong Foundation is a small silicone gel band. It's about as wide as a fingernail, thick enough not to break easily, and is worn as a bracelet. The rubber is colored yellow, like the *maillot jaune*. Pressed into it are letters spelling LiveSTRONG. It was invented in 2004 by Nike's ad agency.

People make a small donation to the foundation, usually a dollar, and get one of these bracelets. These bright wristbands are worn as a motivational device for people recovering from cancer, or their friends and family. The foundation has sold over 40 million of these bracelets worldwide.

The donations the foundation receives aren't all as small as a dollar. In 2006, Armstrong donated $500,000 of his own money to the foundation. He's one of several wealthy people who are making substantial donations to this and other charitable foundations. Bracelets in other colors are being sold by other charitable foundations to sponsor their own programs.

CIVIC DUTY

Austin is one of the fastest-growing communities in the United States. Over the last 20 years, it's changed. It used to be a college town where a young Lance Armstrong rented his first place of his own from J. T. Hoyt. Now it's a hub of high tech with an infrastructure that's scrambling to catch up with the needs of a growing population.

In 2003, Armstrong was disappointed by the crowds of traffic on many of his favorite local roads for training rides. Not as many kids were riding around on their bikes as he remembered they used to when he was growing up in Plano. He came to realize that the city of Austin needed to make some changes. What brought it home for him was teaching his own kids to ride. "We ride around together on the street here," he told journalist Ian Dille, who has become a friend. "But if my kids told me they wanted to ride the mile to school, I don't know that I'd let them."[8] When the nation's most famous cyclist has to drive his kids to school because he's afraid to let them ride their bikes, changes have to happen.

Austin's master plan for bicycles has been updated by the Street Smarts Task Force. In 2007, the task force sent out a letter signed by the mayor and by Armstrong, urging citizens, cyclists, health care professionals, engineers, and urban planners to join the effort to make Austin a better place for people to use bicycles. Their plans have the approval of the city council. The changes include the Lance Armstrong Bikeway: a six-mile route connecting east and west Austin. There's real potential here for spreading the economic benefits of high-tech business and development into neighborhoods that need renewal. These changes aren't about Armstrong himself; they're all about people using bikes. He is just one of the people working to change Austin's infrastructure. His efforts are part of the process of making human-powered transportation practical in that sprawling city.

While he's recognized everywhere he goes when home in Austin, Armstrong isn't mobbed. Not everyone is a fan, not even among the hard-core racing cyclists. They're doing their own things. An article in *Bicycling* magazine quoted Austin cyclist Teresa Nugent: "You read more stuff about Lance on our local racing forum [txbra.org] when he shows up to a training ride than when he's in the Tour."[9]

FIGUREHEAD FOR A NATION

As a professional cyclist, Armstrong is older than the average rider. Most of the top cyclists retire before their mid-thirties. Through 2008 to 2010, his return to racing showed that he could still keep up with the peloton of professionals but that he is past his personal prime.

There are other fields where he is now finally becoming old enough to be treated as a serious contender. One of those possible careers is as an elected official. If Armstrong had run for office right after his recovery from cancer, he might have been elected as a local official or to the Texas state legislature. That might have been as far as he could have gone. With the experiences he has had as a father, an investor, and an athlete with two successful comebacks, he would make a good candidate for higher office.

As a young man, Armstrong would not have been anyone's first choice for higher office. He was both shy when he didn't know what was expected in a situation, and brashly confident when he thought he did know. It took several interviews before he became at ease speaking with reporters. As for speaking in front of a crowd, Armstrong would usually thank everyone and sit down. Only after winning the Tour de France several times did he gain some grace in front of crowds and microphones. It took practice. This talent was worth learning, and gradually he did learn it.

Through his motivational speaking, Armstrong has become familiar with speaking to crowds and media audiences. As the spokesman for the Lance Armstrong Foundation, he has worked with government officials to promote public health through the foundation's programs and activities. He tries to keep informed about new research in cancer and new programs to help people affected by it. This knowledge means that he is not just parroting the words scripted for him by speechwriters. It seems that he has an authentic wish to do good things to help people. As well, he has learned the virtues of having good staff and good associates, each with their own duties to support their collective goals. It doesn't hurt that along the way, he has earned a fortune through hard work and superior effort as well as good luck.

The timing of Armstrong's second comeback could not have been better. As the American national economy was undergoing a reassessment, this trim, athletic man made a good figurehead for renewal. Loren Mooney, editor of *Bicycling*, commented on his timing: "At the critical moment when we as a nation needed a collective comeback, Armstrong returned, older but still larger than life, to lead the charge."[10] She wouldn't be surprised to see him run for Texas state governor and win. Mooney believes he has already been a figurehead for national renewal, through personal example.

INCREASED TURNOUTS

The Lance Armstrong Foundation released a video about the LiveSTRONG Challenge on its Web site in March 2009 and found more response than usual for that time of year. Armstrong told *Bicycling* magazine in 2009 that he believes more people are joining fund-raising rides these days because these rides are fitness goals. Also, people feel like they're making a personal difference in the fight against cancer.

"The Lance Armstrong Foundation has been fortunate to have an increase in our rider/runner/walker numbers in years past," he commented. He doesn't have a number in mind for participation or fund-raising goals. "When it comes to each person, helping out doesn't even need to have a monetary value. Volunteering at a rest stop during a ride can be as rewarding as raising the minimum [pledges] for a ride entry." At rest stops, volunteers hand out water, sports drinks, and sometimes energy bars to competitors. In Armstrong's opinion, the best way to help a foundation event is by going to the event as a volunteer. "It's great to sponsor someone and write a check, but to actually be there and see the event happening is a far better experience."[11]

Money isn't everything to this man. He gave his name to a foundation that raises millions of dollars each year to ease the suffering of people with cancer and to research a cure. His goal is to help other people as he was helped. When his own cancer diagnosis came, friends and family rallied around him in support. Armstrong had expert doctors and nurses giving him the most effective treatments they knew. All this support still wasn't enough, because a person with cancer can feel alone and vulnerable. Not everyone is as lucky as he was. Knowing this, Armstrong supports the foundation's efforts. Together, he and the foundation are trying to help how people feel. Feelings are hard to measure in dollars and cents.

GLOBAL CANCER AWARENESS

Armstrong had a goal in mind when announcing his comeback in September 2008. He wanted to make his return to professional racing part of an international initiative by the Lance Armstrong Foundation. The idea was that he would race in countries that were a focus for the campaign to increase awareness of cancer around the world.

As a writer pointed out for the *Guardian* at that time, "To date the foundation's work has taken place primarily in the United States. Over $260 million has been raised in the pursuit of improvements in the prevention of cancer, quality of life for survivors, the provision of screening and care and investment in research. But now the foundation wants to have an impact worldwide on the stigmas, misconceptions, and lack of awareness on the subject that exists."[12]

Media attention for his training and racing activities were opportunities for Armstrong to remind people about the foundation and the programs it supports. "Armstrong prominently wore Live-STRONG gear and talked up the cause on his Twitter feed and in his homemade videos,"[13] reported *Bicycling* magazine. He spoke with leaders from Australia, Ireland, Italy, and other countries. Riding in the Tour Down Under in Australia was an overall success. Even though Armstrong didn't win the race, he knew the networking and publicity paid off. The Australian health minister pledged to add millions of dollars to the Australian program for cancer treatment and research.

The president and CEO of the Lance Armstrong Foundation, Doug Ulman, is a cancer survivor himself. In 2010, he was honored to be one of many international representatives making presentations at the World Cancer Congress. He was also elected to the board of directors for the Union for International Cancer Control. The foundation is a part of the worldwide effort to understand this disease and to help people who have it.

SEEN IN PASSING

The LiveSTRONG message inspired some interesting ideas. One of these was a clever new invention from the Nike corporation. It was nothing to do with shoes or sportswear. One of their design teams created a machine to write words on a road surface. It could be used to print messages on a road, to be read by participants on the course of a road race.

"Via this device, dubbed the Chalkbot, people could send shout-outs to loved ones dealing with cancer or in remembrance of those who had passed away from it," Armstrong wrote in *Comeback 2.0*. "As we rode, we got to see these good wishes and be reminded of the LiveSTRONG message."[14]

The invention of the Chalkbot is a response to some angry messages that were painted on the roads for several of the Tour de France races where Armstrong was competing. "EPO Lance" and "Armstrong pig" were two of the least offensive of some of these demotivational messages. There were positive messages also, but as Armstrong has commented, one person booing is louder than 10 people cheering. The Chalkbot allows many more people access to the race routes for their positive messages. Chalk is more temporary than paint, worn away quickly by weather and wheels.

"I saw my message on telly as the peloton rode over it," an Australian fan posted on the LiveSTRONG blog. "BIG excitement and doubled when I got the confirmation email so I knew I wasn't dreaming."[15] The Chalkbot words seen in Elizabeth Kreutz's photos show messages that range from upbeat to poignant: "For my mom the survivor," "It's about time to live," "In memory of jean smith;" "George S. you will beat this!" Through use of the Chalkbot, people are able to participate together in the LiveSTRONG program in a way that is still very personal.

CORPORATE SPONSORS

The sponsors who sign contracts with Armstrong do more than give him money to use their products in public and while racing. Oakley is one of the corporate sponsors who stuck with him while he was treated for cancer. This corporation has been a supporter of the Lance Armstrong Foundation from its beginning.

Oakley's product lines include a LiveSTRONG version of most designs of their sports sunglasses. $20 from the purchase of any of these LiveSTRONG products goes directly to the Lance Armstrong Foundation. Over 15 years, the Oakley corporation has been proud to raise over $5 million for the foundation through these products. Other sponsors have products of their own that generate donations for the foundation. Events organized by the foundation are supported on many levels, from small local businesses hosting modest events to large corporate donors.

The Lance Armstrong Foundation joined forces in 2010 with Trek, the maker of Armstrong's bikes. For that season Armstrong and his Team Radio Shack teammates rode on bikes carrying the names of cancer survivors from around the world. The goal was to pay tribute to uncelebrated heroes, and to raise awareness of just how personal the fight against cancer can be.

NEW NIKE VIDEO

During the 2010 Tour de France, the Nike corporation filmed Armstrong on a stretch of steep road in an area called Jura. This mountain would be the final climb for stage 7 of the race. The video was for a new TV spot for the LiveSTRONG campaign for the Lance Armstrong Foundation. The spot was posted on the LiveSTRONG Web site with other news about Team Radio Shack, along with a still photo from the video.

In this video, there's not much color on a gray day. Armstrong is on his bike, pounding up a mountain road. He soars past valleys while the voiceover plays one quiet voice after another. It's as if viewers get to hear all the distracting thoughts of everyone who has faced cancer and turned to a bike or sports and the natural world to recover.[16]

The effect is unifying. He's not the only one overcoming adversity. He's just one of those doing it where his efforts can be seen.

NOTES

1. Lance Armstrong, press conference, October 8, 1996, Lance Armstrong Story, http://autobus.cyclingnews.com/results/archives/oct 96/lance.html.

2. Mary Oliver, "The Summer Day," in *New and Selected Poems* (Boston: Beacon Press, 1992).

3. Lance Armstrong with Sally Jenkins, *It's Not About the Bike: My Journey Back to Life* (New York: Berkley Books, 2001), p. 159.

4. Lance Armstrong, "For Stacy," LiveSTRONG blog, July 20, 2010, http://livestrongblog.org/2010/07/20/for-stacy/.

5. Paula Johanson, *Frequently Asked Questions About Testicular Cancer* (New York: Rosen, 2008), p 53.

6. Bill Gutman, *Lance Armstrong: A Biography* (New York: Simon Pulse, 2005), pp. 113–14.

7. Lance Armstrong, "Lance Armstrong Quotes," BrainyQuote.com, http://www.brainyquote.com/quotes/authors/l/lance_armstrong.html.

8. Ian Dille, "The Local Lance," *Bicycling*, August 2009, p. 66.

9. Ibid.

10. Loren Mooney, "The Art of Lance," *Bicycling*, August 2009, p. 16.

11. Bill Strickland, "Driving Force," *Bicycling*, June 2009, p. 76.

12. Mikey Stafford, "Armstrong Now Pedals to Proselytise as Much as to Win," Guardian.co.uk, January 16, 2009, http://www.guardian.co.uk/sport/2009/jan/16/lance-armstrong-foundation.

13. Bill Strickland, "The Comeback Report Card," *Bicycling*, October 2009, p. 50.

14. Lance Armstrong, *Comeback 2.0: Up Close And Personal* (New York: Touchstone/Simon & Schuster, 2009), ch. 4.

15. Lindy Rol, comments to "For Stacy," LiveSTRONG blog.

16. Nick Shuley, "Video: Lance's New LIVESTRONG Spot," Team Radio Shack, July 9, 2010, http://www.LiveSTRONG.com/teamradioshack/news_video-lances-new-LiveSTRONG-tv-spot/.

Chapter 9

PLANS FOR THE FUTURE

In 2011, Lance Armstrong is going strong. He isn't one of the forgotten celebrities about whom people say, "Where is he now?" or "Is he still alive?" Lance Armstrong is a household name in sports, in the cancer community, and among motivational speakers.

He keeps an exhausting schedule. In any month of the year, Armstrong has several speaking engagements through the Lance Armstrong Foundation. He'll also be meeting with government officials at many levels, from ministers of health to city councilors. As well, he'll be on his bike for races, for charity rides, or for training. Sometimes he takes a bike out just for the pleasure of a social ride with a friend, with a little trash-talking race to the top of the next climb. His physical activities are well described as "cross-training," including everything from hiking to yoga. He likes the University of Texas Longhorns and enjoys hanging out at their football games.

"You know when I need to die?" Lance wrote in his biography *Every Second Counts*. "When I'm done living. When I can't walk, can't eat, can't see, when I'm a crotchety old bastard, mad at the world. Then I can die."[1]

MARATHON RUNNING

Armstrong has never completely left behind his origins as a runner and triathlete. In recent years, he has participated in marathon runs in Boston and New York City, finishing with very respectable times for any athlete.

The New York City Marathon is televised live online through a Web site called TheFinalSprint.com. In 2006 the television crew kept a camera following Armstrong for the entire race, showing him as the race progressed. There are reports that being aware of this dedicated camera kept Armstrong on pace throughout the event. Instead of taking a few moments at points where he would normally have felt comfortable stopping to stretch, Armstrong kept on moving.

Running this marathon wasn't merely a personal goal, it was also a fund-raising campaign for the Lance Armstrong Foundation. Finishing the run earned $600,000 in pledges for the foundation's LiveSTRONG program. His friends Lewis Miles and Robert McElligott ran with him. As well, Armstrong set up a pace team of runners with Nike's help: Alberto Salazar, Joan Benoit Samuelson, and Hicham El Guerrouj. These trained experts kept Armstrong going at a pace intended to help him complete the marathon in a time of three hours. For the last five miles or eight kilometers, Armstrong pushed harder than he'd been going and finished the run with a time of 2 hours, 59 minutes, and 36 seconds. He was the 856th runner across the finish line, but in a field of thousands of runners that is a fine finish. It was a difficult race for Armstrong, who found it harder than competing in the Tour de France. Shin splints were more of a problem than he expected. "For the level of condition that I have now, that was without a doubt the hardest physical thing I have ever done," he said. "I never felt a point where I hit the wall. It was really a gradual progression of fatigue and soreness."[2]

The next year, 2007, Armstrong was able to dedicate more time to training for the New York City Marathon. He was the 232nd runner across the finish line, with a time of 2 hours, 46 minutes, and 43 seconds. He ran the Boston Marathon on April 21, 2008, finishing in the top 500. With a time of 2 hours, 50 minutes, and 58 seconds, he showed the kind of dedication and results seen in trained marathon athletes. At the age of 37, he was performing among the best of the masters class.

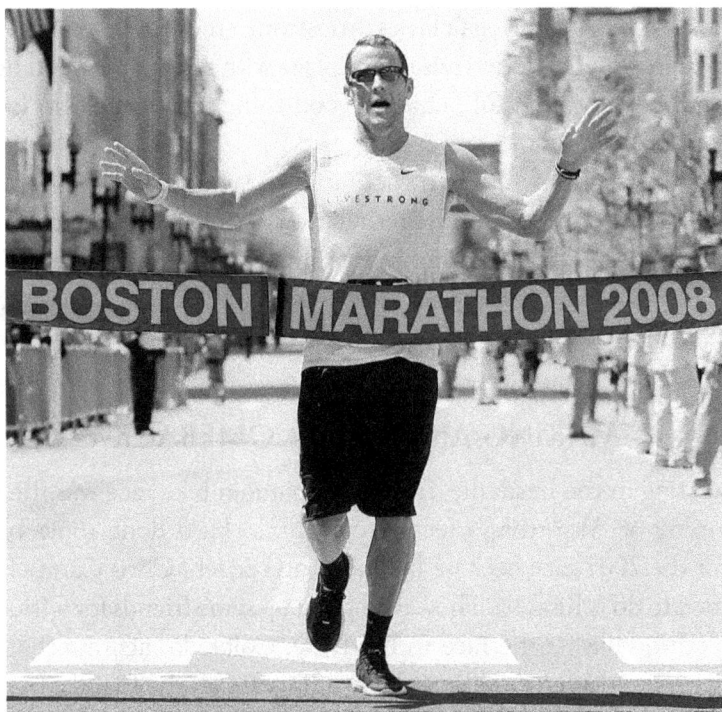

*Lance Armstrong crosses the finish line during the Boston Marathon,
April 21, 2008. (AP Photo/Michael Dwyer)*

OTHER FITNESS ACTIVITIES

In 2007, Armstrong was part of a group of professional athletes who
launched a new charitable foundation. Some of the athletes in at the
start were Muhammad Ali, Warrick Dunn, Tony Hawk, Jeff Gordon,
Andrea Jaeger, Mia Hamm, Jackie Joyner-Kersee, Andre Agassi, Mario
Lemieux, Alonzo Mourning, and Cal Ripken Jr. Athletes for Hope is a
charity that helps professional athletes get active in charitable causes.
Their goal is to inspire ordinary citizens who aren't professional athletes to volunteer in support of community activities.

One of Armstrong's fitness goals is to compete in the Ironman World
Championship triathlon in Kona, Hawaii. He hasn't entered the Ironman yet, but after bike training in Hawaii he has this particular race
on his wish list.

Other fitness activities he participates in are yoga and hiking. He's
been photographed wearing a weighted vest while hiking up Ajax ski

hill in Colorado. The yoga classes Armstrong enjoys are at King Yoga, a center in Aspen. The exercises take place with music and mood lighting and are very peaceful. That's a good thing for a man who is still competitive.

He also attends his children's activities and cheers them on from the sidelines. Part of the reason he retired from professional bike racing in 2005 was because his children wanted him to be at home more of the time. He tries to be present and active in his children's ordinary lives, not just on special occasions.

MAKING ANOTHER COMEBACK

Competing in the Leadville Trail 100 mountain bike race was the real beginning of Armstrong's second comeback. He'd done some training for the 2007 race because his friend and coach, Chris Carmichael, planned to do it himself. They even lined up some friends for a friendly competition during the race in Leadville, Colorado, figuring that the one with the slowest time would buy dinner for all the friends. But the media noticed that Floyd Landis had announced that he would ride that race. Armstrong didn't like the feeling that journalists were considering him and Landis to be in a personal competition, so he stayed out of the race that year.

For 2008, he was ready. When training with Chris Carmichael, he brought up the idea of keeping in training after Leadville and competing again in the Tour de France. It took some time and discussion before Armstrong confirmed that he had approval and support from everyone whose opinions mattered to him.

First on his list was Kristin, his former wife. As Carmichael reminded him, Armstrong's retirement had been in order to spend more time with his growing children. He couldn't get back into the training, travel, and competition without knowing how it would affect Luke, Grace, and Isabella. Because she was the mother of his three children, Kristin's support mattered to him in many ways, even though they were no longer married. Touched that he asked for her opinion, Kristin cried in relief. She told him she had expected him to say he was going to run for political office. Coming out of retirement would be a lot easier on their children than that!

As for the children themselves, they had only dim memories of earlier Tour de France races, more from what they had been told than from anything they really remembered. Now they were excited by the idea of traveling to France and being there with their dad for all the excitement of training and competing.

With his longtime agent, Bill Stapleton, on his side, Armstrong knew there'd soon be enough time cleared on his schedule for training and all the riders he needed for Team Astana to train with to compete in the Tour de France. He raced for no salary or bonuses from team Astana. Philippe Maertens stepped in as the team's public relations manager. With Johan Bruyneel set to be the *directeur sportif* of the Astana team, Armstrong was ready. Bruyneel even left the Astana squad from Kazakhstan, where he'd been training that country's national team for the 2009 Tour de France. Working together one more time would be more satisfying, Bruyneel confided, than working five years with a new team, even if it had the potential to dominate the Tour.

COULD HE DO IT AGAIN?

There was no way to know for sure if Armstrong could come back and win the Tour again. He gave it a shot. His coach Carmichael had been training other athletes during the past three and a half years. Along the way, Carmichael had learned more about the ordinary challenges faced by cyclists who weren't born with Armstrong's unusually high lactate threshold and VO_2 max. Training sessions of five- or six-hour rides weren't necessary for every day. Carmichael had learned that intervals of high-intensity riding during a training session lasting one or two hours had a powerful effect on fitness. In months, Armstrong had restored his physical fitness to the level of the professional peloton.

The sports media and his competitors were much less polarized into either adoring or scorning Armstrong than in the past. "This time around Armstrong seems more likeable by the fact that he's no longer a winning machine," wrote Loren Mooney in an editorial for *Bicycling* magazine. "He is also more inspirational—not just to those affected by cancer, but now also to those of us who may have let ourselves slide for a few years but still dream of staging a stunning comeback."[3]

"In some respects the winning-or-losing aspect of it doesn't matter as much now," wrote Armstrong in his third memoir, *Comeback 2.0: Up Close and Personal*. For him, continuing to dream his dream is what matters most. He wants to imagine challenges and take them on. He wants to try his best. Let the chips fall where they may. "You don't have to have been near death to know that that's what living is all about—but maybe it helps."[4]

After training in Austin, he competed in several races in Colorado near Aspen. Shortly after the 2008 race in Leadville, he raced in Snowmass. Participants can race as three-man teams or solo riders in this local event, called Twelve Hours of Snowmass. His girlfriend, Anna Hansen, competed as an individual rider in this exhausting race. Armstrong rode as part of a team with two local riders, his friends Max Taam and Len Zanni. His team won the event, but Armstrong considers his girlfriend's solo ride for the 12-hour event to be more remarkable.

UNEXPECTED COMEBACK

Completing the Snowmass event solo was not the only remarkable thing about Anna Hansen, as far as Armstrong was concerned. It was at about this time that she conceived his fourth child. It was an unexpected and very happy event for the couple, and for the rest of their family.

It was particularly unexpected because until that moment, Armstrong and his doctors had assumed that he was sterile. His children by his ex-wife, Kristin Richards, had been conceived via in vitro fertilization using sperm that he had put in a sperm bank during the first week of his cancer treatments. While nearly all of the men who survive treatment for testicular cancer are still potent, about a third of survivors are made sterile by the radiation and chemotherapy treatments.[5] Fertility does return for some survivors, and this apparently happened for Armstrong.

The result was little Max Armstrong, born in 2009, a welcome addition to the extended family. Luke, Grace, and Isabella were thrilled to have a little brother.

A year later, Armstrong was proud to tell family and friends that his fifth child was expected. To the many fans following him on Twitter,

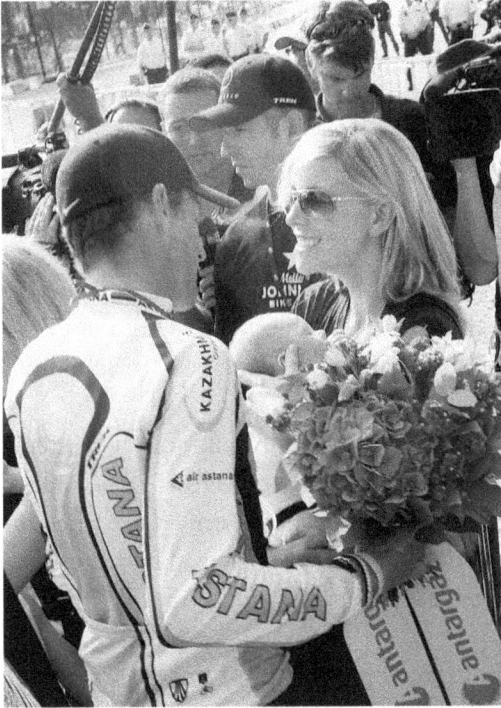

*Third place overall, seven-
time Tour de France winner
Lance Armstrong, left, is
greeted by his girlfriend,
Anna Hansen, right,
holding their son Max, as
he steps down from the
podium after the 21st stage
of the Tour de France
cycling race, July 26, 2009.
(AP Photo/Christophe Ena)*

Armstrong sent out the word that he and Anna Hansen were expecting another child in the fall of 2010. Nicknamed Cinco (Spanish for five) in the womb, this little one was named Olivia.

WRITING ANOTHER MEMOIR

Armstrong's return to competitive cycling is considered to have begun seriously in January 2009. As a friend who was participating in Armstrong's return to training for competition, Elizabeth Kreutz brought up an idea. She wanted to make a book of photographs about this second comeback to professional racing.

Making a book chronicling in photographs the progress of his second comeback was something that might not have occurred to Armstrong on his own. After all, few people under 50 years old have already written two memoirs. He has also been a cowriter on other books about his life events. But Kreutz's incredible work as a photographer was inspiring. Writing captions for her photos became an opportunity to share his work and life in a new way. As a professional photographer, Kreutz has seen her work in magazines such as *Sports Illustrated* and *Newsweek*. She covered five Tours de France and two Olympics. If anyone could help Armstrong make the memories of this comeback into a new and exciting book, it would be Kreutz.

Finding a new way to share elements of his life was an eye-opening experience for Armstrong. He had confidence in his friend Kreutz, and in her work with the camera. It was an effort, but he allowed her access that no other photographers had. She was able to show him not only on the winners' podiums, but also training, playing with his children, and working for the foundation.

Three of Kreutz's photographs were used as inspiration by contemporary artist Shepard Fairey. Best known for his powerful "Hope" image of Barack Obama, Fairey had a new idea. Using a similar style, he created a mural now on display in downtown Los Angeles. There are three panels, with the words "Defiance," "Courage," and "Action!" written above images of Armstrong.

One of the photos that Kreutz took just a day or two before the start of the 2009 Tour de France shows Armstrong's legs as he stands next to his new time trial bike. The bike itself is beautiful as a sculpture or modern art, and Armstrong calls its designer, Marc Newson, an artist. But the cyclist's legs are sculpted, too—as finely detailed as the bicycle that is honed to a micrometer tolerance. Another photo shows him on the start ramp for the Tour. In both shots, under his skin, his legs are well muscled without being bulky, and his calves are wrapped in a roadmap of veins. As Armstrong commented, "Clearly those legs were ready to race."[6] That's the kind of photograph that tells the story of his second comeback.

APRIL 2009 IN SPAIN

Racing in Europe again was exciting for Armstrong. In Italy, he and several members of team Astana rode the Milan–San Remo race on a beautiful day. From there, they went to Spain. He'd been looking forward to the Vuelta a Castilla y León. This was the first time that he and Alberto Contador would be in the same race, and they were even both on the Astana team.

During the first day of the Vuelta, some riders crashed, and Armstrong was caught behind them. There was no room to go around them before he crashed, too. This collision sent him over his bike's handlebars. If he'd landed on his head, it's possible that he could have broken his neck again. But he landed on his right shoulder instead. Team doctor Pedro Celaya was on the case right away, soon joined by doctors at a Spanish hospital. They took X-rays of the injury. The diagnosis was easy: his collarbone was broken into at least four pieces.

A marker has been installed at the place where the crash occurred. "Residents of the village of Antiguedad have erected a monument there," reports *Bicycling* magazine, "which consists of a stone, a plaque reading 'La Clavicula de Armstrong' and a blue-and-white city bike."[7] Such roadside shrines are common in Spanish-speaking countries. Shrines are usually simpler and set at the sites of car crashes causing deaths.

Armstrong's right arm was wrapped in a sling for the long flight back to Texas. Back home in Austin, Armstrong met the surgeon who would repair his collarbone, Dr. Doug Elenz. During surgery, Dr. Elenz used 12 screws to put the collarbone back together. Those titanium screws will be part of Armstrong for the rest of his life. He'll set off metal detectors at airports. In hospitals, he'll never be able to have a magnetic resonance imaging scan again, or the titanium might move. After the surgery, Dr. Elenz sent Armstrong home with strict instructions: don't even think about riding for a week.

The less-than-perfect patient didn't really take to heart that rule about no riding for a week. Two days after surgery, he hopped onto a stationary bike while Anna was out running errands. Before long, the SteriStrip tapes were removed from his healed incision. It was time to get back to training so he could compete in the Giro d'Italia.

At his home in Aspen, he was soon out riding in tricky weather. One April day would be sunny and 75°F (about 24°C), yet the next morning there would be snow on the ground. He couldn't let worry about slipping in the wet snow keep him off the bike. "If you worried about falling off the bike, you'd never get on,"[8] he has said. Snow made for a good opportunity to take his children Luke, Grace, and Bella to Aspen Highlands for beginners' ski lessons. They skied while their dad rode the snowy mountain roads.

STILL HEALING

The collarbone was still healing while Armstrong competed in a race in New Mexico at the end of April 2009. When a young entrepreneur brought hundreds of giant printed images of Lance Armstrong's face to the Tour of the Gila, Lance was both charmed and freaked out. At five dollars a copy, there were faces of Armstrong everywhere in that New Mexico town that weekend.

Armstrong raced in the Tour of the Gila with his friends Chris Horner and Levi Leipheimer as Team Mellow Johnny's. "The three of us totaled up our age at the race, and realized we had more than a hundred years combined," Armstrong said of Team Mellow Johnny's. "We were proud to clean up over the young guys."[9]

For Armstrong, this race could have been a return in some ways to his old habit of getting in front of the pack, something he used to do before he'd learned to ride as part of a team. Instead, it was an opportunity for him to be out front, in the role of the *domestique* who "pulls" along the team leader who is drafting behind him. "The nature of the race [gave] him the opportunity to sit on the front and set a high, steady tempo for long stretches," wrote coach Chris Carmichael. "Overall, Lance spent more power and energy during Gila stages than he would have sitting in the peloton during longer—and even faster—races in Europe. As a result, being a superdomestique at Gila was great preparation for riding the Giro as a supportive teammate."[10]

GIRO D'ITALIA

It's important for a rider to get along well with the team. For the Giro d'Italia in late April 2009, Armstrong wasn't the leader who would be helped to win by the rest of the Astana team. Coach Chris Carmichael and *directeur sportif* Johan Bruyneel decided that Levi Leipheimer was the strongest rider. For this race, Armstrong was a *domestique*, riding in front and letting Leipheimer draft behind him.

This decision was useful in many ways for the team dynamics. For one thing, the coach felt it would be the best way to develop Armstrong's strength that would be put to use later that season in the Tour de France. For another, it would develop more than one possible leader for Team Astana. There was no point in pinning all their hopes for the season on one rider. That wouldn't be teamwork.

STARTING SYMBOL

At the start of each Tour de France, Armstrong was used to getting a little gift from his friend Michel Gamary, who ran a restaurant outside of Nice, where he used to train. These gifts were just little tokens that he could carry with him while riding. But by the time of Armstrong's second comeback in 2009, Gamary's restaurant had been sold, and they had lost touch. There was no way to contact Gamary. But at the presentation in Monte Carlo before the race, Gamary showed up unexpectedly. He told Armstrong that the next morning at 10 a.m., he would come by the hotel with the traditional gift.

This time, it was something like the little metal objects the Spanish call *milagros*. "It was a small gold fish that he had blessed by an Italian priest," Armstrong recalled. "I really appreciated his effort and kept this talisman with me for the entire Tour."[11] He carried this little charm as well as the cross he wears to remember Stacy Pounds.

PULLING FOR CONTADOR

Was it failure when Armstrong didn't win the 2009 Tour de France? Not at all. Finishing this challenging stage race could never be called failure. He wasn't the *Lanterne Rouge* finisher in last place, either. Even after three and a half years of retirement, he was a serious contender to win.

He finished third in the 2009 Tour, behind Andy Schleck in second place. The winner was Alberto Contador, his Astana teammate. Though Armstrong and Contador had not worked seamlessly on Team Astana during this season, for this race in particular, they made serious efforts to work together. At times, Armstrong rode in front of Contador, "pulling" the other cyclist along for part of a stage, allowing him to recover strength by drafting close behind.

Finishing third was a disappointment to Armstrong after seven consecutive wins, but it was not a reason to quit. The experience hadn't soured him on cycling—it gave him new perspective. "For one thing, my legacy—whatever it is—can't be worth much if a lesser result would somehow tarnish it,"[12] he said in *Comeback 2.0.* For another thing, he had plans for the coming year for the Lance Armstrong Foundation and for racing. The 2010 Tour de France was on his schedule.

THE 2010 SEASON

For Armstrong, the 2010 season consisted not only of racing, but of traveling to promote the foundation. He kept a running commentary going on Twitter and Facebook for over 2.5 million followers interested in social media and his activities. Often there were hundreds of comments in reply to each of his updates. Attendees at luncheons might thank him for the motivational speech, or suggest cheerfully that the next morning's local bike ride be done at a social pace. When he mentioned the death of his grandfather, Paul Mooneyham, on August 24, he received over a thousand brief responses.

This year, his team's major sponsor was Radio Shack. Levi Leipheimer and other teammates stayed with Armstrong and *directeur* Bruyneel and Coach Carmichael. Alberto Contador continued to race for Team Astana as the their lead cyclist.

It wasn't only hardcore cycling fans who were turning out for the major races. Impressive numbers of people turned up for races wherever Armstrong went that year. There were tourists and families with umbrellas for shade. Some of the diehard sports fans showed up in costume. On some routes the viewers lined up along the road curbs, often two and three deep for the entire day's ride. "Can someone do the math? How many people are there if it's 225 km and 3 deep? Thanks Holland and Belgium for coming out!!" Armstrong posted on Facebook using his iPhone on Sunday, July 4, 2010. Previously, these kinds of attendance numbers had been seen only for key stages during Armstrong's sixth and seventh victories of the Tour de France.

During this season's races, nearly all of the cyclists competing with Armstrong were younger than this 38-year-old father of four. He raced in the 2010 Tour de Suisse and made a respectable showing among the finishers. At least three of his rivals in that race were the sons of men who competed with him in the past.

Before the 2010 Tour de France, Armstrong let it be known that this was the last time he would be a contender in this race. He was a strong rider in the GC for the early stages.

In his 13th Tour de France, it seemed that luck had left Armstrong at Stage 8, where Andy Schleck won the day. After at least two falls, Armstrong finished the stage with bleeding scrapes on both elbows and a knee, 12 minutes behind the leader's time. Commentators suggested that he would now become a helper for Radio Shack team member Levi Leipheimer, who finished this stage in eighth place, and help him through to win.

The race concluded with Armstrong riding as a *domestique*. The team with the best average time for the 2010 Tour was Team Radio Shack, even though none of Armstrong's teammates finished first, second, or third.

MORE TO SAY

The future still lies ahead for Armstrong. The average life expectancy for an American man is about 75 years. Since Armstrong turned 39 in 2010, he may have 30 or 40 more years to live. After surviving cancer, every day is a bonus.

He's not sure where the future will take him. Not to the Tour de France again, he's said. But a man who has retired twice from professional cycling might take it up again. Certainly he plans to keep riding in charity events and to keep supporting the Lance Armstrong Foundation and its programs.

For someone who has written three memoirs and many other books about cycling, his life, and his foundation, Armstrong still has a lot to say. He was working on an autobiographical film project in 2010. The best place to look for future works about Lance Armstrong is to look for future works written *by* Lance Armstrong.

NOTES

1. Lance Armstrong with Sally Jenkins, *Every Second Counts* (New York: Broadway Books, Random House, 2003), p. 21.

2. "Lance Armstrong: A Classic Case of Too Much, Too Soon." TheFinalSprint.com, January 7, 2007, http://www.thefinalsprint.com/2007/01/a-classic-case-of-too-much-too-soon/.

3. Loren Mooney, "86 Miles With Eddy Merckx," *Bicycling*, October 2009, p. 10.

    4. Lance Armstrong, *Comeback 2.0: Up Close and Personal* (New York: Touchstone/Simon & Schuster, 2009), Introduction.

    5. Eric Huyghe, Tomohiro Matsuda, Myriam Daudin, Christine Chevreau, Jean-Marc Bachaud, Pierre Plante, Louis Bujan, and Patrick Thonneau, "Fertility after Testicular Cancer Treatments," Wiley Inter-Science, http://www3.interscience.wiley.com/cgi-bin/fulltext/106600 998/HTMLSTART.

    6. Armstrong, *Comeback 2.0*, ch. 5.

    7. "Hubbub: Long Live Lance's Clavicle," *Bicycling*, August 2009, p. 28.

    8. Lance Armstrong, "Lance Armstrong Quotes," BrainyQuote. com, http://www.brainyquote.com/quotes/authors/l/lance_armstrong. html.

    9. Armstrong, *Comeback 2.0*, ch. 3.

    10. Chris Carmichael, "From Diesel Truck to Sports Car," *Bicycling*, August 2009, p. 42.

    11. Armstrong, *Comeback 2.0*, ch. 5.

    12. Armstrong, *Comeback 2.0*, introduction.

Appendix

SPORTS AWARDS AND LANDMARK RACES

1984   Fourth in Texas state swimming championships, 1,500-meter
        freestyle
1987   Tri-Fed (former name of USA Triathlon) champion of Texas
        Triathlon magazine's Rookie of the Year
1988   Tri-Fed champion of Texas
1989   Competed in World Junior Cycling Championships in Mos-
        cow
        National sprint-course triathlon champion
1990   National sprint-course triathlon champion
1991   Settimana Bergamasca
        Finished last in the Clásica de San Sebastián
        Second in the Championship of Zürich
1992   First Union Grand Prix
        GP Sanson
        Olympics in Barcelona; placed 14th in road race
1993   Trofeo Laigueglia
        Ninth in the Paris-Nice seven-day stage race
        Thrift Drug Classic
        K-Mart West Virginia Classic

U.S. Professional Cycling National Championship
World Professional Cycling Road Race championship in Oslo,
Norway

1994   Thrift Drug Classic
        Second in Tour DuPont
        Second in Clásica de San Sebastián
        Second in Liège-Bastogne-Liège

1995   Clásica de San Sebastián
        Tour DuPont

1996   La Flèche Wallone
        Tour DuPont
        Olympics in Atlanta; placed 6th in time trial and 12th in road
        race
        Union Cycliste Internationale: World Number 1 Ranked Elite
        Men's Cyclist

1998   Rheinland-Pfalz Rundfahrt
        Cascade Classic

1999   Tour de France
        ABC *Wide World of Sports* Athlete of the Year
        United States Olympic Committee (USOC) Sportsman of the
        Year
        ESPN/Intersport's ARETE Award for Courage in Sport (Pro-
        fessional Division)

2000   Tour de France
        Grand Prix des Nations
        Grand Prix Eddy Merckx
        Olympics in Sydney, Australia; won bronze medal in individual
        time trial
        Prince of Asturias Award in Sports
        World's Most Outstanding Athlete Award, Jesse Owens Inter-
        national Trophy
        Laureus World Sports Award for Comeback of the Year

2001   Tour de France
        Tour de Suisse
        USOC Sportsman of the Year

2002   Tour de France
        Grand Prix du Midi-Libre

Sports Illustrated Sportsman of the Year
Associated Press Male Athlete of the Year
USOC Sportsman of the Year
Presidential Delegation to the XIX Olympic Winter Games

2003   Tour de France
Associated Press Male Athlete of the Year
BBC Sports Personality of the Year Overseas Personality Award
ESPN ESPY Award for Best Male Athlete
Reuters Sportsman of the Year
Laureus World Sports Award for Comeback of the Year
Sports Ethics Fellow for the Institute for International Sport

2004   Tour de France
Tour de Georgia
Associated Press Male Athlete of the Year
ESPN ESPY Award for Best Male Athlete
Trophée de l'Académie des Sports

2005   Tour de France and announced retirement
Associated Press Male Athlete of the Year
ESPN ESPY Award for Best Male Athlete
ESPY Award for GMC Professional Grade Play Award

2006   ESPN ESPY Award for Best Male Athlete
Honorary Doctorate of Humane Letters, Tufts University

2008   Announced return to professional cycling at age 37

2009   Placed third in the Tour de France, riding with Team Astana

2010   February 4, 2010: World Cancer Day
Finished Tour de France, riding with Team Radio Shack

FURTHER READING

Armstrong, Lance. *Comeback 2.0: Up Close and Personal.* Photographs by Elizabeth Kreutz. New York: Touchstone/Simon & Schuster, 2009.

Armstrong, Lance. *The Official Tour de France.* London, UK: Weidenfeld & Nicolson, 2004.

Armstrong, Lance, with Sally Jenkins. *It's Not About the Bike: My Journey Back to Life.* New York: Berkley Books, 2001.

Armstrong, Lance, with Sally Jenkins. *Every Second Counts.* New York: Broadway Books, Random House, 2003.

Armstrong, Lance, with Graham Watson and Robin Williams. *Lance Armstrong: Images of a Champion.* 2nd edition. Emmaus, PA: Rodale Books, 2006.

Barry, Michael. *Inside the Postal Bus: My Ride with Lance Armstrong and the U.S. Postal Cycling Team.* Boulder, CO: VeloPress, 2005.

Bicycling, http://rodale.com.

Bradley, Michael. *Lance Armstrong.* Tarrytown, NY: Benchmark Books/ Marshall Cavendish, 2004.

Bruyneel, Johan. *We Might As Well Win: On the Road to Success with the Mastermind Behind Eight Tour de France Victories.* New York: Houghton Mifflin, 2008.

Byrne, David. *Bicycle Diaries*. New York: Viking, 2009.

Coyle, Daniel. *Lance Armstrong's War: One Man's Battle against Fate, Fame, Love, Death, Scandal, and a Few Other Rivals on the Road to the Tour de France*. New York: HarperCollins, 2005.

The Green Life. Sierra Club website, http://sierraclub.typepad.com/greenlife/.

Gutman, Bill. *Lance Armstrong: A Biography*. New York: Simon Pulse, 2005.

Hurst, Robert. *The Cyclist's Manifesto*. Guilford, CT: Falcon Guides, Globe Pequot Press, 2009.

Hylton, Thomas. *The Bicycle Book: Wit, Wisdom & Wanderings*. Hardwick, MA: Satya House, 2007.

Kelly, Linda Armstrong, with Joni Rodgers. *No Mountain High Enough: Raising Lance, Raising Me*. Waterville, ME: Thorndike Press, 2005.

LiveSTRONG Blog, http://livestrongblog.org/.

Pedal Magazine, pedalmag.com.

Picker, Primero. *Tour Johnny's Tour de France Travel Planner*. http://letourtravel.blogspot.com.

Vélo, www.velomagazine.fr.

Vélomag, www.velomag.com.

VeloNews, http://velonews.competitor.com.

Velovision, http:velovision.co.uk.

Wheatcroft, Geoffrey. *Le Tour: A History of the Tour De France*. London, UK: Simon & Schuster, 2005.

Wilcockson, John. *Lance: The Making of the World's Greatest Champion*. Philadelphia: Da Capo Press, 2009.

Wilcockson, John. *23 Days in July*. Philadelphia: Da Capo Press, 2005.

Yates, Richard. *Ascent: The Mountains of the Tour de France*. San Francisco: Cycle, 2006.

INDEX

About the Author

PAULA JOHANSON has worked as a writer and editor for 20 years. Her nonfiction books on science, health, and literature include *Jobs in Sustainable Agriculture* and *World Poetry: Signs of Life*. Her novel *Tower in the Crooked Wood* is available in print and as an ebook. She was shortlisted twice for the Prix Aurora Award for Canadian Science Fiction Writing, while raising gifted twins on an organic-method small farm. An accredited teacher, she has edited curriculum educational materials for the Alberta Distance Learning Centre and eTraffic Solutions. Johanson rides a Norco Parklane delta tricycle and owns six kayaks.

www.ingramcontent.com/pod-product-compliance
Lightning Source LLC
Chambersburg PA
CBHW050229270326
41914CB00003BA/625

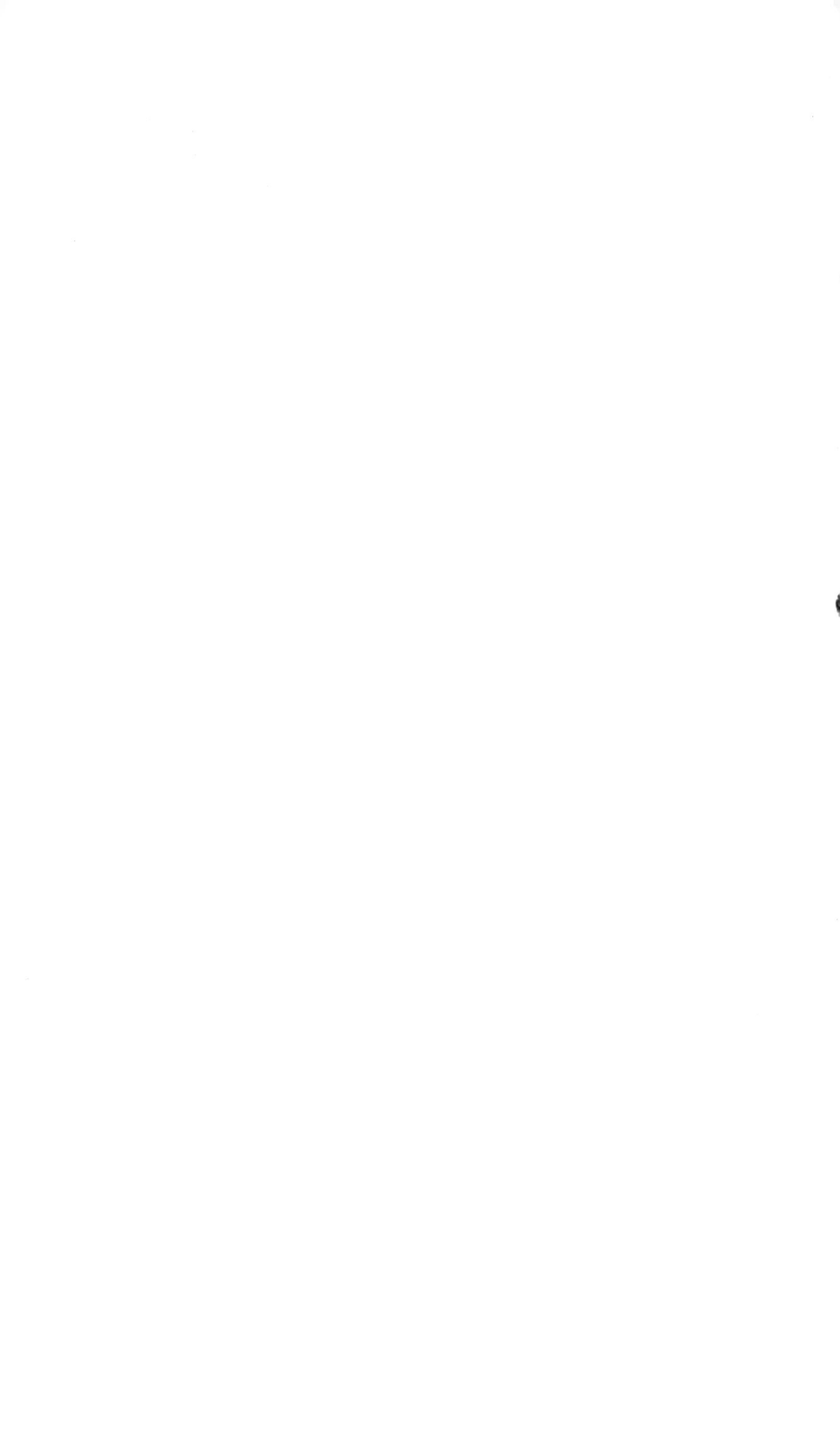